Dr. Jack's Dog Facts

Dr. Jack's Dog Facts

A Guide

To Common

Canine Ailments

by
JOHN BLOXHAM, D.V.M.

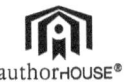
authorHOUSE®

AuthorHouse™ LLC
1663 Liberty Drive
Bloomington, IN 47403
www.authorhouse.com
Phone: 1-800-839-8640

© 2014 John Bloxham, D.V.M.. All rights reserved.

No part of this book may be reproduced, stored in a retrieval system, or transmitted by any means without the written permission of the author.

Published by AuthorHouse 06/26/2014

ISBN: 978-1-4969-2135-2 (sc)
ISBN: 978-1-4969-2136-9 (e)

Library of Congress Control Number: 2014911056

Any people depicted in stock imagery provided by Thinkstock are models, and such images are being used for illustrative purposes only. Certain stock imagery © Thinkstock.

This book is printed on acid-free paper.

Because of the dynamic nature of the Internet, any web addresses or links contained in this book may have changed since publication and may no longer be valid. The views expressed in this work are solely those of the author and do not necessarily reflect the views of the publisher, and the publisher hereby disclaims any responsibility for them.

DEDICATION

This book is dedicated to my sweet wife, Beth, without whose loving encouragement, motivation, and nagging this book would not be.

Also, to my beloved daughter Christian, who typed, corrected, scolded and molded this to completion.

My gratitude goes to the beauty on the cover, Crystal Jackson, of Williamsburg, Virginia, for giving me a big slurpy kiss, and to all of my patients over the years that instilled the idea in me to write this epistle. An indelible reminder that the dog is man's best friend!

FOREWORD

This book is intended to be a ready source of helpful information concerning the more common disease conditions of dogs, gleaned from over fifty years of veterinary practice experience. These are not all of the afflictions, by any means, but those most commonly presented in the clinics and hospitals on a daily basis. The reader will be addressed, and information given, just as if bringing your dog into my office or inquiring by telephone.

Please understand that any type of medical or veterinary 'practice' is not an exact science with many variables, as opposed to the profession of architecture which is more exact. We doctors are allowed our opinions, our trials, and our errors. Some patients survive that were expected to die, and we have all lost those we expected to pull through. You will find differences of opinion from the ubiquitous internet information to your own veterinarian. If you were to take your pet with an issue, to ten different veterinarians, you would probably end up with five or six different opinions! There are often no absolutes in diagnosing and treating illness.

A deep love of animals was birthed into me. My mother loved all animals, so we were well supplied with dogs and cats throughout my formative years. By age twelve, I knew I wanted to be a veterinarian. So this became my dream. I have always believed that my patients should be treated with the least amount of discomfort, and the least expense to the owner. The desired result is a 'waggy' tail, a smiling face, and owner with pets *willing to return*!

John Bloxham, D.V.M.

My pre-veterinary studies were at the University of South Carolina and Clemson University. I graduated from Auburn University's Veterinary School in 1954.

My experiences have varied greatly, having worked for other doctors in three states, in about forty hospitals, including five emergency clinics. Also, I have established five small animal practices in Virginia over the years.

The challenges involved in opening a clinic in a new area gave me great satisfaction. The end result of these many years of experience are presented in the statements and opinions in this book.

It is my sincere hope and belief that the lover of dogs will find this to be the helpful guide to impart the knowledge intended.

John C. Bloxham, DVM
A.K.A. "Dr. Jack"

CONTENTS

Chapter One: The Head 1
   A. The Nose 1
   B. The Eyes 2
   C. The Ears 7
   D. The Muzzle 9

Chapter Two: The Neck 11
   A. Throat Infection 11
   B. Lymphoma 11
   C. Salivary Cyst 12
   D. Slipped Disc 12

Chapter Three: The Chest 13
   A. Emphysema 13
   B. Bronchitis 13
   C. Lipomas 14
   D. Adenomas 15

Chapter Four: The Back 16
   A. Intervertebral disc protrusion 16
   B. Calcified Intervertebral Discs 19
   C. Spondylosis 19
   D. Tumors of the Back 19
      a. Lipomas. 19
      b. Papillomas 20
      c. Sebaceous Gland Cysts 20

Chapter Five: The Forelegs 21
   A. Fractures 21
   B. Strained Muscles and Ligaments 21
   C. Dislocation of the Shoulder or Elbow 22
   E. Lick granuloma 22
   F. Toe Nails 23

Chapter Six: The Hind legs 24
   A. Hip Dysplasia 24
   B. Luxating Patellas 28

 C. Anterior Cruciate Ligament (ACL) 28
 D. Coxofemoral luxations (Dislocated hip joints) 30
Chapter Seven: Anal Glands 32
Chapter Eight: The Skin 34
 A. Flea bite Allergic Dermatitis 34
 B. Tick diseases 36
 C. Bee Stings 38
 D. Hot Spots 38
 E. Yeast Infections 39
 F. Mange 40
  1. Sarcoptic 40
  2. Demodectic 40
 G. Pyoderma 41
Chapter Nine: Reproductive Organs 42
 A. Breeding (On purpose or not) 43
 B. Mammary Tumors 46
 C. Pyometra 46
 D. Dystocia 47
Chapter Ten: Internal Organs 50
 A. The Heart 50
 B. The Lungs 52
  1. Bronchitis 53
  2. Canine Influenza 53
  3. Collapsed Trachea 54
  4. Second-hand cigarette smoke 54
 C. Stomach 54
  1. Gastric dilatation-volvulus (GDV) 56
 D. The Liver 57
 E. The Pancreas 58
 F. The Kidneys 58
 G. Urinary Bladder 60
  1. Urinary Calculi 60
  2. Bacterial Infections 60
  3. Tumors of the Bladder 61
  4. Urinary Incontinence 62

Chapter Eleven: Infectious Diseases 63
    A. Parvovirus 63
    B. Canine Distemper 65
    C. Canine Hepatitis 66
    D. Rabies Virus 66
    E. Lyme's Disease 67
    F. Leptospirosis 67

Chapter Twelve: Internal Parasites 68
    A. Coccidiosis 68
    B. Roundworms 68
    C. Hookworms 68
    D. Whipworms 69
    E. Tapeworms 69
    F. Heartworms 69

Chapter Twelve: This and That 70

CHAPTER ONE

THE HEAD

A. The Nose

Ah, the nose ... that strange protuberance at the most anterior portion of your hairy pet's anatomy. As you well know, your dog's nose has many important uses, not the least of which is its use as a poking instrument. Not all dogs, mind you, but, usually the ones who insist on their way. You know, the smarter ones, we like to think. This is usually proven out on the mornings you hope to sleep just a little bit longer, but are abruptly awakened by this blunt object being shoved into your side, or even face. This loving act conveys so many messages through the wireless communication system: "It's a beautiful day!", "Time to get up!", "Feed me!", "Let's go for a run!", "I need to go to the bushes!", "Pat me!", "I require attention!", etc. *You* understand what your beloved canine is trying to tell you.

But wait! Something is different now ... that nose is usually cold and wet, but this morning it is warm and dry. Why is this? And, what does this mean? Before you scramble to call your veterinary hospital for an appointment, please be advised there is no reason for alarm.

If you think that your pooch is running a fever, use a rectal thermometer to determine this. (Rectal thermometers are more accurate than the ear type)

A dog's normal temperature can vary from 99.5 F to 102.5 F which is quite a range so, as doctors, we factor in other indicators. But if you have a sick dog, you will know something is amiss before you use the thermometer. *So, if your pet's nose is moist and cold, or warm and dry, is of no consequence.*

With sick animals, a comprehensive exam will include rectal temperature, respiratory rate, pulse, blood pressure, check of the eyes, ears, mouth and mucous membranes, lymph nodes, blood and urine analysis, perhaps a cardiogram, x-rays, history of food and water intake, etc. But, nowhere on the patient's chart will you find a notation about the nose: it is not an indicator of canine health.

Another frequently asked question concerns what is termed a "**reverse sneeze**". When this is mentioned to a patient's owner, it always evokes a very quizzical look, implying "What in the world are you talking about!?" The explanation is that this pet has a post-nasal drip, and this is the way of clearing the throat. The affected dog extends his head and, with mouth closed, breathes in and out rapidly through the nose, while making this horrible 'skronking' noise. (You'll not find this word in the dictionary. If the reader can find a more descriptive term, go for it!). Anyway, this is the dog's way of clearing his or her throat. If this becomes problematic for the owner, a small dog can be given 25mg (tablet, capsule or liquid) of Benadryl, as needed, to allay the symptoms.

A larger dog can be given 50 mg for a day or two, as needed.

B. The Eyes

In general, the eyes of our four-pawed friends are subject to a number of conditions similar to those of us two-legged folks. Have you ever gotten a wind—blown speck in your eye? Did it bother you? Of course it did! A little pawing may remedy the situation. Sometimes a good rub can dislodge the speck.

"Why is that eye so red? What have you done to yourself!?" If the furry child keeps acting distressed or holds it shut, your baby needs a trip to the vet. The doctor will examine the eye and do an eye wash. If your dog's eye has been damaged, the doctor will use a staining eye drop to show the affected area. It is important not to let eye damage linger. The vet will prescribe medications for the ailment, and they will need to be administered on schedule to prevent further damage.

Another eye condition we often see is **conjunctivitis.** These eyes appear red— the sclera (the white part of the eye surrounding the pupil) may have a blood shot appearance. The membrane inside the lids may be slightly or very red, and the 'third eyelid' is usually equally affected. This is located in the inner (medial) corner of each eye, and contains a lymph gland (called Harder's gland).

Like any lymph gland in the body, the main purpose is to protect its area; i.e. after tonsils have become enlarged, with a throat infection, resulting in tonsillitis. When the infection clears, the tonsils are supposed to return to normal size.

In a similar manner when eyes become irritated, these third eyelid (nictitating membrane) glands will rise up to defend their property. When I examine an eye, using a topical anesthetic, I always check the back side of the swollen irritated glands. Often times, the surface will have the appearance of large grit sand paper—this is diagnosed as follicular conjunctivitis. This condition usually responds well to a combination of antibiotics and steroids, either in ophthalmic ointment or drops. The drops may be easier to instill in the eyes, but will need to be done four times daily, whereas twice daily treatment with the ointment usually suffices. Treatment duration will vary, but I always say to continue the medication until the eyes are completely normal. With the dogs that have been rubbing their eyes, I like to recommend an 'Elizabethan collar' (which all dogs and their owner's hate with a passion!). If the dog has been rubbing his eyes, he will continue to after each time he is medicated. So, the eyes must be protected if the medicine is to do its job.

Conjunctivitis is usually bilateral (both eyes) albeit one eye could be worse than the other. If only one eye is affected, I suspect an injury or foreign body. Possibilities include a cat scratch, or a wound from a thorn, or thick brush (especially in hunting dogs). Again, using a few drops of topical anesthetic, once in a great while, a grass awn or even a cut blade of grass will be discovered lurking beneath the lower lid.

A **wound in the cornea** (the pupil portion of the eye) can be dangerous and very painful. What appears as a puncture is referred to as an ulcer. The depth of this wound will dictate the healing ability and how long and what medication must be used. With any wound of the cornea, therapy is twofold: prevent pain and infection while waiting for the tissues to heal. Often this is easy, sometimes very difficult. "The book" says corneal tissue should replicate itself in seven days.

My treatment regimen consists of using atropine (drops or ointment) to keep the pupil dilated, thus relieving pain, and antibiotic ointment to prevent infection. And of course, the dreaded "Elizabethan collar". This is usually prescribed for seven days and then I re-examine the eyes. If the wound is healing nicely at that time, I may stop the atropine, and add a steroid to the antibiotic and re-check again in another week. The goal is for complete healing with as little scarring as possible.

I have had some patients return for the first re-check, and had to glance at the chart to remind myself which was the affected eye; It had healed so beautifully! By the same token, I've seen other patients on re-check and just 'crawled all over' the owners for not following my simple instructions because these affected eyes were not one bit improved! After their soulful pleading that they had followed my instructions to the letter, I had to apologize and accept the fact that 'the book' was not entirely accurate, that not all corneas heal in seven days.

Referring to the third eyelid gland, sometimes called Harder's glands, I feel compelled to set forth the following: When these are chronically enlarged and protruding from the corner of the eyes, these are commonly called **"cherry eyes"**. This condition can be seen in any breed at any age. Until about forty years ago we were all cutting these things out, just removing them with no consequences. Then about thirty –odd years ago, some ophthalmologist got the bright idea that these glands should not be removed, but, instead, turned under and secured with a permanent suture. The supposed theory was that later in life, in the eye whose gland had been removed, that this could become a 'dry eye', that there would be some interference with normal tear production. This was taught in all the veterinary schools since the latter 1970's. To this I say, "Hogwash!" I believe that dry eyes come from an anatomical defect. I have seen so many over the years that still had their third eyelid glands. Moreover, in over fifty years of removing these glands, I have yet to prove that a dog has developed a dry eye, years later, in that eye alone. The lacrimal glands in the upper eyelids are also responsible for producing tears and keeping the eyes moist.

Throughout my experience, I have watched countless veterinary surgeons tuck under these eyelid glands as they were taught, using permanent sutures. In many instances, in a month or two, these sutures will give way and the affected gland would pop right up again.

When the pet is returned to their doctor for an explanation, the only one given is, "I'm sorry; this sometimes happens". The offer is made to re-operate to repeat the procedure, and usually for the same fee! I've talked to owners who have had the procedure done twice, and sometimes to both eyes. After the glands pop up again in a few months, the owner admits, "I can't afford to keep having this done!" As a result, you will frequently see a Shih-Tzu or a Cocker Spaniel with cherry eyes, wagging his tail throughout life, but apparently not finding a clinician willing to remedy the situation by simply surgically removing those ugly things. To me, this is a shameful disservice to the pet and an insult to the owner!

Another eye condition frequently seen in small white breeds is **excessive tear stains** from both eyes. The tears show pink to brown on white hair. There is no medication to prevent this, but there is an excellent product for removing the stains, called 'Angel Eyes'.

Another eye condition that is just as common in dogs as in older people is **cataracts**. This condition is a progressive opacity of the lens, and gives the lens a cloudy appearance. There is probably some inherited gene factor contributing to their formation, but also the ubiquitous free radicals can be the major cause, just as with us human types.

There is no magic age at which we begin to see cataracts. The dogs are almost always geriatric and a slightly cloudy mist appears in both lenses as early as ten years of age, although most are in their teens by the time the condition is quite obvious. When I first observe cataract formation on routine exams, I caution the owner to not let their hairy beloveds drive after dark.

At times, **juvenile cataracts** will be seen, especially with a disease like diabetes. It is indeed pitiful to see a two year old dog completely blind. Cataracts can be easily operated, just as with people. The surgical fee is what prevents most owners from having the procedure done. The going rate by an ophthalmologist is anywhere from one to two thousand dollars, plus, per eye. If only one eye is operated, this will allow the pet to live a normal life.

Cataract surgery should have been taught to all students in vet schools. The procedure is relatively simple but very intricate, and a surgeon needs to develop skill for this. This is why most clinicians will refer eye surgeries to the veterinary ophthalmologists, usually found in larger cities.

Glaucoma is also seen in dogs as with humans, and is just as hereditary. The intra-ocular pressure in eyes is checked with a "Tonopen", a human instrument that is fairly accurate. These instruments cost several thousands of dollars and not every practitioner has one. This is something that should be done because glaucoma can easily lead to blindness. The normal pressure, measured at the front of the cornea, is between 14 and 28 mm Hg. If the pressure builds higher over a period of time, it destroys the optic disc in the back of the eye, affecting the optic nerve, resulting in loss of vision.

When glaucoma is diagnosed, human eye medicines are used to keep the pressure within normal limits. This is a life-long treatment, usually twice daily. The eye drops most commonly used are 'Timolol', and are not necessarily expensive.

Should eye pressure be very high (over 40 mm Hg or so) a small tablet can also be given, called 'Methazolamide'. This is a small generic tablet. All eye medications are by prescription only. The Methazolamide, is a carbonic anhydrase inhibitor, which helps prevent the formation of intra-ocular fluid. This also is usually given twice daily if needed.

Another eye condition seen often is **entropion** which can affect both eyelids, but more commonly the lower lids. This is very common in Chows, Sharpeis, Rottweilers, and sometimes individuals of other breeds. This is observed in puppy hood and will always cause trouble sooner or later. The problem is the eyelid turns in and under, constantly brushing against the cornea and is an annoying condition. The only treatment is surgical correction, and this is easily accomplished by every practitioner.

We commonly see small tumors of the eyelids in middle age to older pooches. The majority of these are on the lower eyelid. These are **benign adenomas**. In the beginning, one looks almost like a small tick on the edge of the eyelid. But they always grow larger over time. As the tumor grows larger on the outside of the eyelid, the roots are also growing thicker on the inside of the lid, causing chronic irritation with every movement of the eye. This is why I recommend early surgical removal of these growths.

This procedure is simple, and necessitates a 'v' shaped incision all the way through the lid in order to completely remove all of the root system. If done properly, the eyelid should heal beautifully with little or no scarring and the procedure should not be expensive.

Speaking of tumors, there is another one which is commonly seen called a **histiocytoma.** Although this has nothing to do with the eyes, I simply mention it here because these are usually found around the face. Histiocytomas can be found anywhere on the body but most often they will be seen around the head, face, and ears. These tumors are small, round, and bright pink to red in color. They are sometimes called a "button tumor", referring to the shape. They are always benign and never spread. They seem to pop up almost overnight. Except for their ugly appearance, they do no harm. Should a dog scratch at one, it may bleed a little.

Now, "the book" says if you will leave them alone, some day they will drop off just as suddenly as they appeared. In my "book", I don't want to have to look at this ugly thing on my beautiful dog for two or three or four months before the stupid thing decides to disappear. So, I advocate early surgical removal which is very simple, and my dog is beautiful again (or handsome—as the case may be)!

For the poor beasts that are permitted to ride half way out a car window, while moving at 50 of 60 mph, I can only shake my head in disbelief and utter a phrase like, "Some people don't have the sense God promised a Billy Goat!"

Why don't these owners ride with *their* heads out the window, with no eye or ear protection? What a crazy suggestion! Yet if you question the owner as to why they allow their pets to do this, the reply is always, "He loves it so!"; which, again brings up the question of intelligence. (I will allow the reader to jump to his/her own conclusions, because, I can already sense the arguments to my remarks even before this manuscript goes to print!) A couple of years ago, I saw this motorcycle with a side car. Riding in the side car were two dogs, one a Beagle and the other a Lab type, both wearing eye goggles! They were thoroughly enjoying the ride with good eye protection. I would like to have conversed with the cyclist but was unable to do so.

C. The Ears

Problems with dog's ears are probably the most common conditions seen, second only to skin diseases. To make matters worse for many canines, their ear conditions are related to a skin disease, so that treatment for one has to include the other. The most common of these are various allergies that affect different areas of the body and often including the ears. (Dermatalogical conditions will be discussed further in the chapter on skin).

The most frequent signs that an owner might observe will be shaking of the head (less common), scratching at or rubbing the ears (most common), accompanied by a bad odor from the affected ears. As the owner inspects the ear, the canal is usually filled with blackish gunk, and there may be inflammation of the skin surrounding the ear canal. This is called, **otitis externa** and is extremely common.

The causative agent is usually bacteria and /or yeast (which is a fungus). Many vets will make a smear onto a slide, from the gunk, to examine under the microscope to be able to see what type of bacteria and/or how much yeast is seen. For treatment of these ears, the ear canals have to be cleaned GENTLY!

All the gunk is removed in order to determine if the ear drum (tympanic membrane) is all right, or might it be ruptured? If the latter is true, this dictates all of the ear medicine that *cannot* be used, leaving only a few that are not ototoxic (harmful to the ears) and may be safely used. Fortunately, those perforated ear drums *do* heal, usually in seven to ten days, and then the ear prescription can be changed. I always choose one that covers both bacteria and yeast, with a steroid to relieve poor Napoleon's inflammation. And, he won't like it, of course, but we have to use an Elizabethan collar or some device to protect his ears so he *absolutely* cannot scratch or rub them while the ear drums heal.

Ear mites are not nearly as common as most owners think. Seen more in puppies, these little bugs come from the mother and are transferred during her mothering. Dogs can get these from contact with other dogs. Usually with ear mites, the dogs will shake their heads more than they will scratch at their ears. Whereas with ear infections they will do more scratching at their ears than the shaking of their heads. Ear mites are very easily treated; let your veterinarian give you the proper medication for your pet.

Dog's ears have cartilage in the middle, covered with skin, and many small blood vessels between. When a dog's ear flap is injured by some type of bruising, one or more of these little blood vessels is broken, resulting in bleeding between the cartilage and skin.

By the time the pet's significant other notices something amiss, the poor ear flap is all swollen. There doesn't seem to be any pain, but probably feels funny because many dogs will shake their heads or they scratch at this grotesque ear in an attempt to make it all better.

These are called **aural hematomas**, and your veterinarian must perform a corrective procedure. There are many methods for this, and we each have a favorite procedure with which we have obtained the best results. After this has been done properly, the ear flap usually regains its normal appearance. If the procedure is not done well, a "cauliflower ear" will be the result. Hearing is not impaired; only the appearance is affected, which means no more movie offers!

D. The Muzzle

The mouth that is home to that long, pink appendage that licks anything bacterial (or worse!) and then your face contains ten more teeth than you. You brush your thirty—two teeth at least twice daily, perhaps more, and what about your four-legged child? It would be wonderful indeed if our canine children would let us brush their teeth at all, but precious few have been trained to do this. So, we have to rely on our family vet to inform us when Fifi's teeth need to be cleaned. We refer to this as a 'dental', short for dental prophylaxsis. Let your doctor show you the purpose in regular cleaning; don't wait for years until some of the teeth have gotten so bad that they have to be extracted. "Preventive health" is the watch-word.

Ordinary bacteria in the mouth are aerobic bacteria. But, when **calculus** (tartar) builds up on teeth over a period of time, these bacteria, now under the surface, have become anaerobic. These can spread to the heart, liver, or kidneys and contribute to their downfall with no prior warning. This is one reason I consider preventive dental care to be so critical, and not just for a cosmetic smile, as we humans tend to think. Some breeds, especially smaller pooches like Miniature and Toy Poodles and Yorkies, are prone to get tartared teeth faster than large breeds, apparently regardless of their diet. If you are the proud companion of a smaller breed of canine, please pay close attention to his or her teeth; so, when you get licked in the face, the halitosis doesn't bowl you over!

Permit me to express my opinion of the several oral preparations on the market for cleaning teeth: these are definitely helpful in removing the tartar that you can see, but bear in mind they do nothing for any anaerobic bacteria just underneath the gum line. Your dog could still have some periodontal disease even though the teeth appear fairly clean. Here again, please go by your veterinarian's recommendations.

While we are on the subject of teeth, for you owners who allow your best friends to chew on wood—a stick, or anything—sooner or later you will experience a foreign body stuck between teeth. Again, your friendly family veterinarian can remedy the situation very easily and painlessly, and your pet will be forever grateful. However, the memory will wane with the next stick he finds. Oh, the joys of parenthood!

There is one condition of the muzzle that is frequently misdiagnosed, resulting in a disgruntled owner. A dog may be presented with a firm swelling perhaps an inch in front of an eye, on the muzzle. At times, the swelling will erupt and exude pus. Antibiotics are given with immediate improvement.

Alas, a few weeks later, there is recurrence requiring further measures. I have seen a few doctors cut into these swellings, and probe around, then suture up the wound, give a different antibiotic and expect different results. All, to no avail.

The problem stems from an **abscessed tooth**. Our canine friends are so stoic; they will not let us know when they have a tooth ache. Only after they chew their food on one side over a period of time, can we determine that there is a bad side. Most frequently, I have observed the described condition in a middle aged dog whose teeth appear quite normal. So, it is only after a particular tooth –in this case it is the upper fourth pre-molar (or carnasal tooth) — is extracted that we see a permanent cure.

This type of abscess would be seen on a dental x-ray, but there is nothing else that causes what I have described. I don't understand how some folks mis-diagnose this fairly common condition. But again, we vets are all "practicing", aren't we?

CHAPTER TWO

THE NECK

A. Throat Infection

Dogs have several sets of lymph glands (nodes) in the neck and under the throat, as we human creatures do. Very commonly, whenever a pooch develops an **infection of the throat**, these glands will enlarge as a matter of course, as part of the body's defense mechanism to fight off this foreign invader. These can easily be seen in a slick haired dog like a Dachshund.

Palpating these, as in all lymph glands, is part of our normal physical examination. Ordinarily, enlarged lymph glands will gradually return to normal once the offending infection has been done away with. Occasionally, one particular gland may remain larger than normal for a period of time. These we re-check periodically and, eventually, they, too, will diminish in size.

B. Lymphoma

Infrequently, dogs will develop **lymphoma** (Hodgkin's disease) causing every lymph gland in the body to become grossly enlarged and hard. It is indeed a sad sight to see one like this. These dogs become anemic and weak over time. A veterinary oncologist may offer some hope with chemotherapy. In general, this may prolong life for three to six months. As with any type of cancer, the owner must make decisions based on the best advice available. There are new treatments (one from Texas A & M) that show promising results and may bring more hope.

C. Salivary Cyst

There is an infrequent condition of the throat that will be mentioned here, what is commonly called a **salivary cyst**. This is a soft swelling filled with saliva, usually due to a blocked salivary duct. They are non-painful and cause no trouble, they just look ugly! If the saliva is drained out (by a big syringe or cutting into it), the cyst will soon be full of saliva again. Usually a veterinary surgeon will decide on the best course of action in order to effect a cure.

D. Slipped Disc

Sometimes I wish there were laws requiring a person to pass an intelligence test before acquiring a puppy. A case in point was a beautiful Great Dane pup, maybe five months old, with a very painful neck. The poor beast was trying to keep from having to move his head. When I laid my hand on his neck, the muscle spasms from pain were so obvious. The owner had just a regular collar on him, and I readily discerned the cause of the problem. In trying to train this pup, the owner had yanked hard on the leash, jerking the collar enough to cause an intervertebral disc to rupture in his neck! This condition is referred to as a **"slipped disc"** by most of us. This most often occurs in the back, especially the lumbar area, both in dogs and in humans.

Every patient is different and responds differently to various treatments. My absolute favorite is a Class 4 laser. This is usually used every other day for three times the first week, twice the second week and once the third week. This works wonders for most disc patients and can be repeated as needed. This is much less expensive than surgery and gives better results sooner. Along with this laser treatment, meds to relieve pain and muscle relaxants are also used.

Chiropractic may be useful early to help relieve pain, but the laser therapy cannot be beat for long-term relief, in my opinion. Unfortunately, these lasers cost a great deal, so very few practitioners have them.

Skin problems of the neck will be discussed in Chapter 8.

CHAPTER THREE

THE CHEST

A. Emphysema

Some years ago, when I was working for another veterinarian, an older lady came in one morning with her Pekingese with an eye problem. As I bent down to examine the face, I was taken aback by the manner in which the dog's breathing was labored, rapid and shallow. Hastily applying my stethoscope, all over both sides of this little Chinese chest, I turned to the lady. As gently as I could say the words, I informed her that her beloved pet had **emphysema**! I inquired if anyone smoked in the house, and she readily admitted that she did. There was just she and her little dog in the house. She burst into tears and said she'd never smoke in the house again! Sorrowfully, the damage had already been done. For twelve years this innocent little being had been inhaling second hand cigarette smoke. His lungs (and hers) were hopelessly ruined forever!

Treatment for emphysema is extremely limited. A veterinarian may recommend something that may be a little helpful for breathing, but officially there is no effective 'cure'.

B. Bronchitis

Bronchitis is a very common condition of all breeds, of any age. It can occur by itself, or as a result of some pulmonary infection, even pneumonia. Anyone who has ever boarded his or her dog is familiar with the "kennel cough shot" that is required before boarding. Since any immunization takes a period of time to develop immunity in order to provide protection, unless a pet had had a previous one within six months, the pooch may not have adequate immunity. Many times a dog will start coughing after arriving home from the kennel, and the owner wonders, "Why?"

For treating bronchitis, I will use antibiotics and suggest a human cough syrup containing dextromethorphan (DM), recommending a child's dose for a small dog and an adult dose for a Cocker sized dog or larger. As with people, this is an excellent preparation for allaying the symptoms of a cough. (More on bronchitis can be found in Chapter 10 under "Lungs").

C. Lipomas

These are tumors consisting of only adipose (fat) tissue. They can be found anywhere on the body, but occur primarily on the chest and abdomen. They are always soft, well-rounded, and you can get your fingers around them. As with most tumors, they begin small but always grow. And grow they do! I removed one that weighed four pounds from the chest wall of a small dog. The dog was about twenty five pounds, so you can imagine how relieved he was after surgery!

I am an advocate of early tumor removal, while they are still small. Invariably, as a few years go by, an owner will present a dog with multiple large lipomas, and discuss questions of age, necessity, what will happen if they are not removed, etc. Mainly, it boils down to how ugly, or uncomfortable, do you want your pet to become? In Virginia Beach, some nine years ago, I saw a big black Lab that had a lipoma half the size of a football! The poor dog was having trouble walking— the tumor was on the chest but under his fore leg. So, with every step, he had to swing his right foreleg out and around this grotesque growth. After the horrible thing was removed, he walked normally with a smile on his face and a wag in his tail!

I suppose this is another area in which I disagree with many practitioners. So many owners have brought their dogs to me for my opinion, long after another doctor had advised them to not worry about a small tumor, "It is not causing any harm". Not then, as a small lump, but down the road it may be quite another story! May I relate an extremely dramatic episode? One Christmas season I wanted to take some time off and contracted with a relief veterinarian to take over my practice for a week. During this time, a client presented his Golden Retriever because of a growth over the spinal column of the pelvis. This doctor examined the tumor, and made a needle aspirate of the interior to check under the microscope. After a short while, the client was told that the tumor was just a lipoma and was advised to "not worry about it".

Three months later, this client retuned with his dog, now having difficulty walking. I naturally informed the owner that what might have been a lipoma is now something far more serious. I referred the owner to our state teaching hospital for a thorough work-up to see if surgery were an option. Unfortunately, this devilish thing was cancerous and had metastasized to other parts of the body, so this poor dog had to be euthanized. Had surgical removal been performed three months earlier, might this pet still be with us? Can you better understand why I am a believer in early tumor removal, while they are still small, and before they become troublesome?

D. Adenomas

Adenomas are usually small, and remain so. They are very firm, non-painful, and are typically smaller than the end of your little finger. They usually appear as a blemish with age, and rarely cause a problem.

Dogs can be afflicted with many other kinds of tumors, much like humans. Those that do become cancerous are infrequent, but occur often enough to question any growth. If your doctor suspects something and wants to do a biopsy, by all means, you want a definitive answer. If the response is good news, does he still recommend surgical removal of a small tumor? Let him or her do it! Preventive medicine is a good watch-word!

CHAPTER FOUR

THE BACK

A dog's back, much like that of its owner's, is subject to similar types of injuries, the worst of which is the very common **intervertebral disc protrusion**, usually referred to as a *'slipped disc'* or a *'ruptured disc'*. Some will just say a patient has a 'disc lesion"—this encompasses a great area. These disc injuries can occur anywhere in the entire vertebral column, but by far, the most frequent area is the lumbar, the lower back. Placing a distant second would be the cervical area, the neck.

Unless a dog has been hit by a car or fallen out of a tree, the owner is usually perplexed as to the cause. Your best friend had not done anything unusual, for him; he has zipped off of the porch hundreds of times to chase a squirrel and it's never bothered him before! It seems as if there is a first time for everything.

This type of injury can occur in probably any breed of dog, young or old, large or small. The cause may be something as simple as jumping onto or off a bed, running down the stairs and missing the last two steps, playing roughly with a larger dog, etc.

One that particularly stirs my memory was a large, handsome, very muscular Boxer whose master would bounce a tennis ball for the dog for their play time. The ball would bounce higher and Brutus would jump to catch it, and then return it to the pitcher for more fun. Well, the ball bounced, Brutus leapt into the air to catch it, apparently, twisting his back. As he crashed to the ground, he could not get up— his hindquarters were paralyzed from a slipped disc. Episodes like this are, unfortunately, all too common.

For the benefit of a reader who may not be familiar with the injury, let me simplify an explanation of what happens. God created us beings with vertebral columns with built in safety features. Our spinal cords run from the brain down to the tail bone in a canal through the tops of all the vertebrae, protected by ligaments and spiny processes of bone. The discs are cartilaginous material placed between each vertebra. I liken these to little, round sofa pillows whose purpose is to allow flexion of the vertebral column, and also to act as shock absorbers. These 'sofa pillows' do an amazing job of fulfilling their purposes under normal circumstances. But when a middle aged man bends over to pick up something heavy without bending his knees, or supporting his lower back, something is going to happen in his back! Those discs are only so strong.

By the same token, if a dog's back is subjected to an unusual strain, a ruptured disc can easily occur. When this happens the 'sofa pillow' bursts at one side, and the cartilaginous material is squeezed out —pressing on the spinal cord— thus the pain and paralysis.

Every case is different, so the treatment and results will differ. The veterinary surgeon that performs spinal surgery, gets pretty good results if he or she can operate within twenty four hours of the injury. I say 'pretty good', meaning 50% to 75% cure rate.

Years ago my daughter had a little Dachshund, named Eva. This dog was such a delight—always happy and full of life. Well, one day her little short legs and long spinal column proved to be her downfall—she did something to injure her back, resulting in a ruptured disc.

I called a colleague, who does spinal surgery, to ask his opinion. He could only give a 50% chance of recovery if he were to operate on her spine. That wasn't good enough for me, so I chose enforced rest with anti-inflammatory tablets. I kept her in a cage in my hospital, taking her outside four times a day to relieve herself, supporting her with my hands.

John Bloxham, D.V.M.

Her hind legs were paralyzed. If I held her in a standing position, her back toes wanted to turn under—a very bad sign. The prognosis did not look good at all.

At the end of the first week, I saw a slight improvement. At the end of the second week, I knew there was definite improvement. After three weeks, she was so much better. At the end of the fourth week, that little badger hound was perfectly all right, and went on to live out her normal life with no more back problems, just as full of zip and zest as before the injury!

Now, I would have to say that Eva's recovery was exceptional. Absolutely every dog with a spinal injury must be treated as an individual case. No two dogs can be compared even though the symptoms may appear to be similar, and even the x—ray views may appear to be equal in injury to the spinal cord, the results of treatment will vary. This is regardless of the kind of treatment used!

Many dogs will improve to a point, but never be perfectly all right. Others may show some improvement but not enough to be pain free, unfortunately. These, at some point, are usually euthanized.

Each veterinarian will recommend what he/she thinks will prove the most beneficial. In the last several years, the class four laser has proven to be a real boon for effective therapy, especially if it can be started early. These instruments are very expensive, so very few veterinarians have them.

The class four laser is used every other day for three treatments the first week, then two treatments during the second week and once during the third week. Conclusions may be assumed after a few treatments. After the third week, if a dog has made an apparent full recovery, the patient can receive a repeat of one or more treatments if needed in the future.

In cautioning owners of spinal injury dogs about after and future care, I say if you have any stairs in your house, to sell it and get a ranch house with no steps. Also, put all sofa cushions on the floor, so everyone sits on the floor. Mattresses also go onto the floor in order to eliminate all possibility of Fido's ever again jumping up onto anything! (Another recommendation is getting a crate for the hapless patient to keep him from climbing and jumping while the family is out).

B. Calcified Intervertebral Discs

Older dogs will frequently develop **calcified intervertebral discs**, over a period of time. The owner usually has no clue of this until there is an episode of spinal pain and posterior paralysis. These will cause the same type symptoms as a younger dog with an acute slipped disc. With the calcified discs the prognosis is nearly always poor, depending on the degree of paralysis.

C. Spondylosis

Another condition of older dogs, as with humans, is **spondylosis** of the spinal column. This is likened to arthritis of the vertebrae—bony bridging build across the ventral surfaces of some vertebrae. There is no pain involved, only stiffness over a period of time. This results in poor posture in people. In dogs, the hindquarters are usually lowered somewhat, and the normal stature and gait are impaired. It just looks like an old dog, standing or moving.

Although, their appearance may be pitiful, take comfort in knowing there is no pain involved, only stiffness. Some physical therapy methods, such as hydro-massage, swimming, etc. may be of some help in keeping old Buster's back a little more limber, but I know no sure—fire way remedy for spondylosis. (Arthritis of the hip joints will be discussed in Chapter 7).

D. Tumors of the Back

a. Lipomas.

Tumors felt on the back of the dog, are usually **lipomas**. These fatty, benign tumors are described in Chapter 3, about the chest. These usually cause no trouble unless they become so enlarged that they keep the dog from resting normally on either side. It is usually best to get these things removed surgically before they get larger than a quarter in size because they always grow larger.

b. Papillomas

Papillomas are quite commom—small and ugly—but do no harm. These are usually seen in middle-aged and older pets, and resemble warty growths. They are benign but can easily be removed surgically.

c. Sebaceous Gland Cysts

These are seen frequently. These are firm, round thickenings in the surface of the skin. As one is firmly squeezed, sebum oozes out and the cyst is no longer a cyst until, after time, it refills with more sebum. These do no harm and are seen on dogs as they begin to age. Usually, I will tell the owner to remind me with each visit and if the **sebaceous gland cyst** needs squeezing, I will do it then. These can be easily removed surgically if the owner desires.

CHAPTER FIVE

THE FORELEGS

A. Fractures

With the exception of dogs having been struck by cars, or some other source of trauma, **fractures** of the canine fore legs are not too common. There are exceptions, such as the slender legged Italian Greyhound and these types of little dogs, whose long, thin bones are looking for trouble.

One very common injury regarding the fore legs happens to puppies being held, then dropped suddenly, by children. We see fractures of the paws and long bones, primarily the radius, from this type of injury. These fractures can also happen when small dogs or puppies fall or jump off a bed or sofa, or sometimes falling down some steps.

Depending on the pup's age and size, some splints will permit decent healing. Implanted stainless steel pins work fine, if the bones are of sufficient age and size.

After-care is always a concern. The children still want to hold the little beast, want to run and play, etc. Healing for bones is slow and must be approached with patience. The patient must be cared for as an invalid, and not as an animated toy!

B. Strained Muscles and Ligaments

Dogs also experience **strained muscles and ligaments** of the shoulder and elbows. Usually, recovery of these injuries is of no consequence as long as the patient can be given enforced rest. This is another situation where crating can be beneficial.

C. Dislocation of the Shoulder or Elbow

Dislocation (luxation) of the elbow is very uncommon, unlike the hip joint. Returning the elbow is done the opposite way of other joints; with every other joint dislocation, the correction consists of extreme extension of the appendage in order for the affected bones to go back into proper place. The elbow is the only exception to this —with this joint it must be fully flexed (under anesthesia, of course) in order to correct the dislocation.

Sometimes we will see a fractured condyle of the elbow (distal humerus). These fractures are repaired with surgical screws.

There are other orthopedic conditions of fore legs that will just be mentioned because they occur more infrequently. Panosteitis and hypertrophic osteodystrophy can both cause acute discomfort and lameness in the long bones of young dogs. Fortunately, both conditions tend to be self-limiting. Your veterinarian will further elaborate.

E. Lick granuloma

A very common malady of the skin of the foreleg, or forepaw, is the **lick granuloma.** I'm sure that the reader is familiar with the old wives wisdom concerning a sore on a dog, "Let him lick it and it will heal just fine". NOT SO!

This is the sole cause of lick granulomas—the sore spot just gets bigger, thicker and uglier. The dog absolutely cannot be allowed to let his nose get anywhere near the affected area. The same rule applies to a cut or sore he can't lick, but can (and will) scratch to a raw, inflamed, and very painful mess!

Various medications have been used with varying results. Whatever protective device can be employed to keep mouth, and paw, separated from sore, will prove invaluable. It will take time, yes, depending on how bad the granuloma appears.

I have operated on some to remove the offensive area to shorten the healing time, provided the owner makes a solemn promise to keep the protective device on Beauregard 25 hours a day, and 8 days a week! This is, absolutely, the only way to effect healing of a lick granuloma.

F. Toe Nails

In regard to toe nails, some large dogs that run around on rough ground and pavement may never need their nails trimmed. But most smaller dog's nails need to be clipped periodically. Really, any nail trimming should only be done by your veterinarian. Not only will it be done correctly, he or she has an assistant that can hold your dog gently but firmly to assure accuracy with the least amount of stress to your dog's psyche. It is worth a trip every three months for this potentially dramatic procedure.

In the mean-time, between visits to the vet, you can use an emery board on nails that grow sharply or quickly. Once again, care should be used that the emery board is not gouging into the pad while sanding the nail tip. Care should also be taken to not pull your pet's foreleg out of joint in order to try to accomplish this. Have another adult hold your pet securely. After doing this often enough, usually pets will tolerate a quick 'tip sanding'— as long as it is rewarded.

If you are giving your quadraped child a pedicure, do not try to cut back to the quick of the nail—always stay away from cutting so close. It is foolish to cause pain and bleeding. Unfortunately, some groomers like to trim nails too short. Apparently, they think the paws look neater. Poor dogs!

CHAPTER SIX

THE HIND LEGS

The hind legs of dogs possess similar characteristics, in anatomy and orthopedic problems, as those of humans. Some people inherit a deformed hip joint (coxo vera and coxo plana) which can be likened to the all-too-common hip displasia of, mainly, large dogs. A dog's stifle joint corresponds to our knee joint, with luxating patellas and ruptured anterior cruciate ligaments.

They may not sprain their ankles (the tarsal joint) like we do, but they do have their share of strained ligaments. Also, the hind leg is the appendage that suffers more fractures. If a veterinary student learned to surgically repair fractures, it was the hind leg that was used in surgery class.

A. Hip Dysplasia

This is an inherited condition that causes the hip joints (coxo femoral) to become deformed as a large breed puppy grows. Sometimes it may appear to be mainly in one joint, but in the vast majority of cases, both joints are usually affected, albeit one slightly more so than the other.

It seems that the German Shepherd breed is most frequently incriminated in discussions of this malady, although any breed larger than a Cocker Spaniel is subject to developing some degree of hip dysplasia. Because of the German Shepherd's popularity, most studies of hip dysplasia have been done with this breed, beginning back in the late 1950's.

These joints are said to resemble cups and saucers; the saucer being the end of the hip bone (acetabulum), and the cup is the head of the femur, the big thigh bone. The ideal acetabulum is like a crater with a smooth surface. The ideal femoral head is full, rounded, and smooth.

With different dogs, we find every conceivable variation and degree of dysplasia—from almost normal to absolutely pitiful. For example, instead of one dog's acetabulum being a well-rounded, deep "saucer", it may become shallow and almost flattened. In addition, instead of the head of the femur being a nicely rounded "knob", it may appear to be anything but this. So, the end result is a very ill-fitting joint, just begging for trouble. As time progresses, the dysplastic joints become arthritic, developing rough, sharp surfaces. This is also termed **degenerative joint disease.**

Since this condition is only diagnosed by use of the x-ray (radiogram), a certifying organization was set up to advise owners who mail in their dog's x-rays. This is The Orthopedic Foundation for Animals, usually spoken as O.F.A.

In order to take a proper x-ray, a dog must be sedated for a short time in order to be properly positioned on the x-ray table. The dog is laid on his back; one person will extend the fore legs and another pulling the hind legs back, and slightly rotating the legs inward. If this is done just right, both knee caps will be super-imposed over their joints. In this manner, the radiologist can be assured the pelvic position will enable the hip joints to be properly exposed.

The O.F.A. requires dogs be at least two years old before submitting their films. I have known some owners of beautiful dogs that are too eager to find out about their pets. Some will request an x-ray at 12 months of age, "Just to see how they look"; other owners may wait a little longer. But regardless of how beautiful the hip joints may appear at that time, dogs can still be developing the malady up to two years of age.

Most conscientious owners will try to obtain a definitive history of both sets of parents—was everyone certified normal by O.F. A.? Even so, this is no guarantee that the progeny will be normal. By using the Mendellian Laws of Inheritance one might be able to determine the chances of any puppy developing hip dysplasia—but which puppy? Whose puppy? No one could possibly know.

Frequently, folks will purchase a large breed puppy from a reputable kennel, make all of the proper inquiries concerning hip dysplasia, or other maladies of large dogs, get their copy of the pup's AKC registration certificate – in short, do all of the needful things before bringing King or Queenie in to the family. They proudly show off and relate the new puppy's pedigree. The mind-set soon becomes one of wanting to replicate this outstanding example of canine perfection. Just look at him or her! What terrific conformation, and coloring and personality, and etc., etc., etc.

As the puppy grows, carefully laid plans are made with regard to breeding. If theirs is a male, they can have first choice of a puppy from a new litter in lieu of a stud fee. If it's a female, speculation is begun on how many pups there may be. Naturally, a dollar amount for profit is always considered. This is a given!

Now, we can see this puppy is far more than just a family pet. As he or she matures, the owners anxiously await the news of "when can the hips be x-rayed"?

Finally, at about two years of age, the family veterinarian says, "Now is the time."

Very often, the hopeful owners are given anything but good news. Even though the parents and grandparents were O.F.A. certified 'normal', this perfect specimen of the canine world is not quite perfect—at least not in the hip joint department!

Now, the big question: Should the dog be neutered? Since hip dysplasia is an inherited condition, and a dominant one at that, in all good conscience, no honorable owner should allow the affected animal to breed. Neuter the male, spay the female, and be done with the anxiety!

There is an alternate method of determining if a puppy is developing abnormal hip joints. This procedure is called the "Penn HIP exam", and is performed at several stages of the growing young puppy. Not all veterinarians are familiar with the Penn HIP exam. The main advantage is being able to advise a puppy's owner before awaiting a full two years for the O.F.A. X-ray procedure.

Now, for the dogs who have developed arthritic hips, there are several available options for treatment. These dogs don't become lame overnight—it takes years before they exhibit signs. Usually, the most obvious is difficulty in getting up on the hind legs from a lying position. This is most noticeable on a slick floor.

From here, the owner sees the lack of agility that has taken place over time. And finally, frequently one hind leg will exhibit more lameness than the other. By this time, the veterinarian has probably prescribed pain medication as well as the chondroitin sulfate—glucosamine tablets. The purpose of this latter preparation is to help stimulate the production of joint fluid, and to hopefully produce cartilage growth for the cushioning in the joints.

For those dogs that are severely lame, the most common surgical procedure for this is the femoral head ostectomy (FHO). Here the ugly, arthritic head of the femur is just removed. A "false joint" forms surrounding the surgical area, and as many months pass, the patient can walk and run much better, even pain free. During this time, some muscle atrophy will occur because Rambo is not yet locomoting normally. Given more time, these muscles will re-develop and the leg will appear quite normal.

For many years, this has been the most frequently used surgical remedy. There is another involving cutting a muscle tendon on the inside of the thigh. The theory behind this is that cutting this tendon relieves pressure on the hip joint. Unfortunately, the method does not work well all of the time.

Now, for folks with very "deep pockets", joint replacement is available just as with people. The big catch is, it is so expensive that very few surgeons are asked to do this type of surgery. Consequently, the owner desiring this would probably be directed to a veterinary school. As with people, with the proper technique by an experienced orthopedic surgeon, joint replacement should last a life time!

Now, anytime we see a lame dog, regardless of the diagnosis, pain medication will be prescribed. Obviously, the critter is hurting or wouldn't be limping. These pain medications are called "NSAIDS", for non-steroidal anti-inflammatory drugs. These are non-narcotic. They act on the nerve receptors where ever there is pain. They do a good job, but have one serious flaw. These drugs can affect any dog's liver. This is why when a veterinarian has a patient on an NSAID for very long, he/she will do a blood panel every six months (if not more often) to see if any of the liver enzymes are elevated. This is the only way to determine ahead of time if trouble is brewing.

We have all heard the horror stories of how Rimadyl— one of the most popular NSAIDs dispensed—has killed dogs in just a few days. Fortunately, these are very few in number compared to the millions of dogs given the drug.

Speaking of pain control please be advised that **no human over-the-counter preparations**, (like Advil, Aleve, Tylenol, Motrin or any brand of ibuprofen) **can be given safely to dogs and or cats!** *It can poison them!*

Now, how best to relieve Fido's arthritic pain? Is there a substance that won't cause any harm, is not expensive, that works like a charm for the most arthritic joints? How about something that is natural? There is such a product called "Lubrisyn". This can be like a miracle— for man and beast.

The active ingredient is hyaluronic acid, which is the precursor of all joint fluid. So, instead of two rough bone surfaces rubbing against one another, they can be cushioned in viscous fluid. I liken this to putting motor oil in an engine that had none. Some veterinarians may carry Lubrisyn.

If not, it can be ordered by calling, 1-800-901-8498. The dosage for man or beast, is one tablespoon daily, regardless of size. For dogs, this can be put directly on their food that would be readily consumed. For two legged animals, this may be mixed with any juice or milk.

B. Luxating Patellas

In small breeds, mainly the toy and miniature types, quite often the knee caps will not stay where they are supposed to, but will luxate, move around to the inside. This position causes interference with the knee (stifle) joint flexing properly. If this is not corrected, in a young dog, the legs will malform, become bowed as the poor little fellow tries to walk and run.

Fortunately, this condition is easily remedied by surgery, without costing a great deal. Some dogs only have one knee cap causing a problem, but invariably the other will follow suit because of such a shallow "trochlear groove" in the lower end of the femur, the thigh bone. We must remember that when man manipulates breeding—for example, the toy and miniature poodles—some deviation from the natural is bound to occur; consequences are to be expected.

C. Anterior Cruciate Ligament (ACL)

This condition has become the number one orthopedic problem with dogs, and I don't know why. Forty and fifty years ago, it was not nearly as prevalent as it has become. Have our dogs' life styles changed that much to cause this?

We used to see more "hit by cars" for many years, resulting in all types of fractures. But this business of Buster shooting off the porch to chase a squirrel, just as he's done a thousand times before, and coming back limping on a hind leg. What did that squirrel do to him?! Or, Hannibal, charging down from upstairs because he heard someone say "car ride", and skipping a few bottom steps, continues running for the door, but now with a limp. Or darling Susie, she always hops up and down to be on the bed. But this time, she jumped down, but went away limping.

With people, it takes a very traumatic injury to cause an ACL to "rupture", such as a football player getting tackled hard. But apparently many dogs just sustain these injuries from their normal activities.

There are two ligaments that cross behind the knee joint (stifle in the dog), thus the term "cruciate". For some reason it seems that the ligament in front (anterior) is always the culprit. Some text books and authors insist on calling this the "cranial" ligament, meaning towards the head. It is exactly the same injury that is so common in athletes, so let's let an ACL be an ACL, and everyone will comprehend.

When the ligament is subjected to undo stress, it breaks—just like a shoe lace breaks. I don't know why the term 'rupture' is used, but one is said to have *ruptured his ACL* and now he is lame. The anterior cruciate ligament enables stability between the femur and tibia, at the stifle joint. So when this ligament is broken, naturally the joint is no longer stable, hence the limping.

The two broken ends cannot be tied or sutured together to effect healing; the ligament must be replaced. There are several methods of doing this. One is to use a strip of muscle fascia from the thigh as a substitute ACL. Probably the more common method of repair is to use a strong nylon fishing line for this purpose. There are other methods and materials, usually determined by the surgeon's success rate with each.

I am sorry to say that canine cruciate repair has gone from several hundred dollars to almost two thousand, depending on geographic locations. Regardless of the method of repair, the aftercare is super important.

Once, in my last practice, I operated on a young Jack Russell's ACL. I really felt good about it. I gave the owners, a young couple, explicit instructions about aftercare, in order for the leg to heal properly. Within two weeks, the couple had gone to visit friends that had a young Lab. Yep! They let the little Jack Russell and the big Labrador play! You know what happened to the leg I had just operated. They returned with their little pup—lame again!

With large dogs, sometimes in order to properly correct the injured stifle joint, it is necessary to perform am orthopedic procedure called a tibial plateau ostectomy. This flattens the head of the tibia in order to better stabilize the joint.

D. Coxofemoral luxations (Dislocated hip joints)

We used to see this type of injury commonly associated with a dog having been hit by a car. I suppose the emergency clinics are still seeing their share.

This can be diagnosed without an x-ray, but sometimes there will be a fracture in the pelvis, so to do a proper job, x-rays are required.

In order to replace the dislocation, a deep anesthesia is imperative. The patient must be completely relaxed because great manipulation is required to relocate the wayward femoral head.

As a rule, if the femoral head slips back into the acetabulum easily, this means it will slip back out just as easily. Wherefore if very great effort and strength are required before success is achieved, this means there is a good chance the joint will stay good.

After the luxation has been corrected the leg is bandaged tightly in a flexed position, emulating an Ehmer sling. If the leg can be kept in this manner for 10 days, the patient can be expected to be "home free", assuming the joint is still normal when the bandage is removed.

It seems that my Ehmer slings always slip or loosen somehow after a few days, and the procedure has to be repeated, making certain that the dislocation is still corrected. For those few who do slip in and out easily, a surgeon will need to perform a specialty operation, in order to provide Rufus with his normal locomotion.

For medium-sized and large dogs, I much prefer to insert a "DaVita pin" to secure the joint. Using this method, we don't bandage the leg in flexion. In order to do this properly, the pelvic x-ray has already been taken and the dog is still under anesthesia from having the joint corrected. The veterinarian will choose a stainless steel intramedullary pin, threaded on one end, the same size that would be used if one were going to pin a femoral fracture.

The DaVita pin should remain for 10 days. Rufus can walk about normally, but activity should still be restricted. If the pin has been placed properly, there is no way the joint can dislocate. The corrected joint capsule and ligaments should be healed, then the pin can be removed. Only very light sedation should be necessary.

I love this method of assuring the dislocation will not occur during healing. This DaVita pin method apparently has become "out of vogue". It is no longer described in text books or taught in schools. I know not why. Unfortunately, only the older veterinarians may know of this most excellent method of solving a frustrating problem. This procedure is easily performed, there is no need to refer to a specialist. This should not be expensive, and certainly would be much less than going to a specialist. The dogs don't seem to be uncomfortable while the pins are still in place. In fact, they want to resume their normal activity and not behave as invalids!

CHAPTER SEVEN

ANAL GLANDS

I don't know why this topic should be deserving of a chapter heading, but believe it or not, this is one of the most troublesome areas of the canine anatomy. Almost every dog at one time or another, sooner or later, will scoot his or her bottom. This is less common in large breeds, but very common in medium and small breeds.

Anal glands are actually small sacs, a pair, one on either side of the rectum. These are the same glands or sacs that skunk's utilize at will for defensive purposes. Not so with dogs. Dogs have no willful control over theirs. Sometimes when a dog is in a fight or injured, the anal sacs will be emptied. The contents can range from a consistency of toothpaste to yucky liquid. It always stinks to high heaven; the odor is very difficult to wash off.

If an owner can learn to express his or her dog's anal glands, the ideal time to do this is when Rocky is in the bathtub and all soaped up. I would still recommend using a rubber glove with a wad of cotton, to prevent a very smelly hand. As I said, the smell is hard to wash away!

Whenever you notice your four-legged companion scooting, the anal glands need to be expressed. Your brother-in-law will tell you that this is a sign of worms. Tapeworm segments can cause an itchy rear, but maybe in 2% of 'scooters' is this the reason. The other 98% of the time it is from the discomfort of the anal sacs feeling full. The poor little beast is attempting to attain some relief by scooting, but, alas, it never helps. Mom, dad, this means a trip to your friendly neighborhood veterinary office. Nothing is to be gained by waiting.

Frequently, we will find an anal sac that is abscessed, and will need to be lanced in order to clean out the bloody, pussy mess. Then, we flush the area with a sanitizing solution and administer antibiotics for 7 to 10 days. Usually healing is uneventful and everyone resumes a happy face.

Some owners allow themselves to become frustrated over the frequency of the trip to the vet whenever Marley starts scooting. I had a sweet Cocker, named Buster, who would scoot just about every 30 days, like he was on a monthly schedule. He would scoot on soft ground, a sidewalk, or even a gravel driveway in an attempt to get some relief.

Some veterinarians will operate and remove the anal sacs if the owner becomes demanding. This will provide a permanent solution, but I just don't like to recommend it. By having Marley come to the office every month, or two, or three, affords me the opportunity to keep up with his general health and weight, not to mention good client relations. I am an animal person, but I'm also a people person. I like to develop relationships with my pet owners, and take a genuine interest in them.

My last practice was in Virginia Beach. One client, a Navy captain, gave my family a personal tour of an aircraft carrier at Norfolk Naval base. Another client, a Navy SEAL Commander, invited my wife and me to a change of command ceremony. Clients who were police officers arranged for ride a-longs in police cars, and several times in the police helicopter! Yes, I enjoy building relationships with clients and taking genuine interest in their furry children's welfare!

CHAPTER EIGHT

THE SKIN

Some dogs seem to never have any trouble with their hide, and others have nothing but problems. These can range from simple flea bite dermatitis (allergy) to pyodermas and chronic yeast infections, with apparently no cure. There seems to be no end to the number of allergens that can affect dogs. Indeed, I would suspect that the average work day of the veterinary dermatologist would have very frustrating moments.

A. Flea bite Allergic Dermatitis

This is one of the most common skin problems of all dogs, but can be readily controlled by diligence on the owner's part. All dogs are allergic to flea bites, just some more so than others.

Since fleas abound in warm weather, we see this disease more frequently in the summer months. The tell-tale sign of this is irritation on the back, beginning at the base of the tail. There will be intense itching, and thinning of the hair with reddening of the skin.

It is not unusual for an owner to exclaim, "But Doctor, I don't see any fleas on him!". Whenever I hear this, I keep looking, using a flea comb, until I can demonstrate at least several fleas.

Fleas constantly move around on their hapless victim; they never stay still. Some dogs can have a "bajillion" fleas, (that's a lot) and scratch some, but may not have any dermatitis. There are others, when assaulted by very few fleas, will break out with the aforementioned skin trouble and act like they've been stung by a horde of wasps!

By this time, fleas are in the house also. Fleas are extremely prolific: one female can lay 5000 eggs in her short lifetime (up to a year and a half!). This is why flea control cannot be a haphazard action; one must go at it with a vengeance!

There are many flea preparations on the market, and the average pet owner can find him or herself in a quandary; which is the best? Who has the best price? Which is easier to use? To whom should I go for the best advice? This is where I must climb onto my soapbox: In an attempt to save a few bucks, we are actually doing our pets potential harm. Here is why . . .

Big-Box-Mart can sell a few pet products perhaps a tad more cheaply than you may think, but whom are you going to ask about what product is best, or can your pet use it? Can your children be around it? Are you going to ask the clerk in the aisle (good luck finding one) or the cashier? But, the only advice they can give is what they do for their pet or their experience with the product. Incomplete advice, at best. You could call 'Pets-a-Million Dollars' (shipping is free and they send a treat for your pet!) and save a few bucks. But, they are not allowed to give pet health advice and what happens if your pet has an adverse reaction to the chemicals in the product!? They can do nothing for you.

A return policy cannot help your dog who may be unconscious and having muscle tremors (a side effect that is possible with some flea preparations). To watch your pet experience adverse reactions is a very scary thing for an owner to experience, not to mention Rover is not having a good time. Time to go to the Animal Emergency Clinic (if you're lucky enough to have one in your area) and hope you get him there in time! The guilt is overwhelming: all in an effort to save a few bucks.

Please know that having your Veterinary office there for you to call with questions, speak to trained staff, and take your pet to see his or her regular doctor ensures the good continued health of your dog. Your pet's doctor cultivates a special relationship with your pet. The doctor cares about the welfare of your pet, knows its history, knows him or her inside and out (literally). This is such a wonderful, local, resource for your communities of pets and pet lovers.

Did you know that approximately 30% of business income in a veterinarian's office is derived from product sales? Did you know that without those sales, many vets would find it hard to stay in business?! Can you imagine if 30% of your family's income disappeared!? Did you know that vets are limited in what they can charge for those products? They cannot 'jack up' the prices to suit them. No, there is a manufacturer's retail price, so there can be no price gouging. In fact, there are many coupon and discount programs in which veterinarians participate in order to pass that savings to the owners, and help with your pet's product costs.

Back to flea control, for treating a dog with a flea bite allergy, I like to give an injection of steroid (usually triamcinolone) to quiet the inflammation and relieve the itching. Now, the control of the fleas is paramount; usually, the owner will agree to both a flea shampoo and then a topical preventive, such as Advantage or Frontline. Sometimes the fleas seem to develop a resistance to one preventive that an owner may be using for their pet. We find that it is best to alternate different products to make it harder for the fleas to become resistant to the chemical in the preventive.

It is also necessary to kill all the fleas in the home, the bedding, the car and the outdoor kennel. Some owners will call an exterminator; others will treat the homes and yards themselves. All of these measures are helpful but it may be necessary to re-apply them often throughout warm weather. Do not stop with flea control even in the winter; as your heating is on, the fleas can live year round inside your home and on your toasty pet. Since eggs can wait to hatch, it will be just that much harder to regain control when the weather warms up.

Many of these exterior flea killing products contain dangerous chemicals and many owners are afraid to use them around their families, and often worry about nature as they treat outside. There are a few natural treatments available, that are effective, but must be used daily or at least every other day. A proactive, multiple hit strategy is a most effective for avoiding a flea infestation every summer. Incidentally, many of these preparations are also very effective on human lice infestations. They work better and are much cheaper than the grocery store nit treatments.

B. Tick diseases

Since ticks are primarily warm weather aliens also let's lump their control with the flea products. All of the good preparations will treat both fleas and ticks. The most notorious tick condition of late is Lyme disease. This was named after Lyme, Connecticut. Although there has been more published about this in recent years, it has apparently been around for many years unrecognized.

Although the deer tick has been named the incriminating vector, other ticks are probably just as guilty. I, personally, do not like ticks. I am a ferocious tick killer, not caring what species or genus one may happen to be.

A Lymes test is easily accomplished from a drop of dog's blood, along with the heartworm test. In Lyme disease, polyarthritis is the most common clinical ailment represented in dogs. Lameness can be acute or chronic, with one or more painful joints. Fortunately, Lyme's usually responds nicely to treatment with doxycycline for three weeks.

Another very drastic condition is tick paralysis, although this is very seldom seen in the clinic situation. This usually happens with an outside dog that apparently has some super sensitivity to tick bites. The patient is brought in panting, lying on his side, unable to walk. In fact, the legs act like "rubber legs" if the dog tries to walk. There may be many ticks, or only one engorged female may be found.

The idea is to kill and remove the nasty creature. When this is accomplished, the result is miraculous. Usually, in less than 30 minutes, the dog is perfectly all right.

As an aside, let me mention an easy way to remove ticks, from people and dogs. Soak a small piece of cotton with white vinegar and hold this onto the tick. It may take a minute or two but the monster will turn loose and not leave much of a sore.

For many years we used various dip solutions for dogs in helping to prevent fleas and ticks. Usually this weekly ordeal worked marvelously if done on a regular schedule.

For a long time there was a product called Dermaton, an organophosphate, which was very effective. In fact, if a dog owner used this every week, fleas and ticks were no problem. We would purchase the Dermaton in one gallon cans, and then fill 3 ounce bottles with it, put our dispensing labels on them, and sell these over-the-counter. The stuff was very potent; one only needed one half ounce, (a tablespoon), to a gallon of water for the dip.

John Bloxham, D.V.M.

One Saturday morning a lady came into my animal hospital with two Dachshunds for some routine task. She inquired about the dip solution and said she'd like to get some. Since she had two dogs she requested two of our bottles. So, I gave them to her and she left. Monday morning, as soon as we opened the office, there was a telephone call from the state Medical Examiner's Office. He asked me, what was the active ingredient in the Dermaton dip that I had dispensed to the lady on Saturday? I envisioned an accidental poisoning, an astronomical lawsuit, etc. Then, the good doctor interrupted my thoughts by saying there was no accident. This woman intentionally drank both bottles of the concentrated dip! What a horrible way to commit suicide! How sad for her pets!

C. Bee Stings

Stinging insects are just as troublesome to our canine children as they are to us. Yellow jackets and wasps are the worst offenders because their stings become so inflamed. Usually, a pet will give a yelp and then jerk around to try to clamp jaws on the assaulting winged creature. Some will carry on more than others, so be prepared to give a generous supply of sympathy in a soothing voice.

In addition, human antihistamines are definitely helpful. Benadryl is usually readily available— a Cocker size and larger dog should have an adult (50 mg) dose, a smaller dog can have a child's dose (25 mg). This is either by liquid, tablet, or capsule. Usually one dose will suffice.

Speaking of a dog's discomfort, never give aspirin or Tylenol, or any ibuprofen, to your dog. Your veterinarian can prescribe pain medication to use as needed and is much safer for your dog. This doctor will determine which is safer for your dog. If it is one that might become harmful to the pet's liver, please heed the doctor's advice on drawing blood samples every six months to be certain that the liver enzymes are not elevated. This is of the utmost importance if any critter is being given pain medication on a fairly regular basis.

D. Hot Spots

The proper term for this condition is "moist eczema". The term "hot spots" accurately describe this most painful of all skin diseases. We see far more cases in hot, humid weather. But they can occur at any time of the year.

This is a surface bacterial infection of the skin, that can be found anywhere on the body or legs. A lesion will begin small and rapidly enlarge. A nickel sized lesion today will be a half-dollar size tomorrow, and if it is in a place the dog can lick or scratch, the following day the lesion will equal the palm of your hand! Not only is the lesion enlarging its borders, it is also growing deeper into all of the layers of the epidermis. And the discomfort is driving 'Cuddles' insane!

Whenever a canine parent sees a small lesion, that is the time to act. Too often one may be noticed on a Friday, but the family has busy plans for the weekend, so the poor pup may be required to wait until Monday morning. By this time the lesion has grown exponentially, and the poor dog may have to be anesthetized in order to properly treat this horrible malady, because it is so painful.

Hair has to be clipped, the lesion cleaned with antiseptic soap solution, then an antibiotic solution. Antibiotics and steroids are given by injection, then antibiotics topically. This area must be protected from licking or scratching. When all goes well, definite improvement is seen on a daily basis, and most of the lesions are resolved in 7 to 10 days.

E. Yeast Infections

This is a very common fungus infection. It is smelly, ugly and just not nice. I believe almost any breed is susceptible to this, but it is more common in some breeds, Sharpeis, Cocker's, Pugs and others. The most frequent area of a dog's anatomy where yeast infections love to persist are the throat, chest, under the forelegs, inside the hind legs, and nearly always the ears. There is a very characteristic odor. The skin becomes thickened and dark. There is usually moisture that is the cause of the odor. In the ears, "gunky" material fills the ear canals. If the gunk is light tan, this usually indicates the cause is mostly yeast. Whereas if the gunk is dark, this usually means bacteria and yeast are present.

There are many methods of treatment, utilizing all types of shampoos and topical solutions (including vinegar), all with varying degrees of success. But, I'm sorry to say, very few are curative. Keeping this obnoxious condition under control may be the best for which the keepers may strive.

The same for people, it is thought that feeding on foods that contain brewer's yeast and baker's yeast (which almost all pet foods do) perpetuate the problem. Trying a yeast free diet is a possible first prevention. There are also pharmaceutical preparations that can act as a fungicide; these have some side effects and some animals cannot use them if they are suffering from other maladies.

If any readers have found excellent success in treating this disease, please contact us through the website in order to share your treatment success. I shall be most pleased to stand corrected. Please continue the success and watch those ears!

F. Mange

1. Sarcoptic

There are two types of mange found in dogs: sarcoptic and demodectic. In humans, the sarcoptic kind is called "scabies". This appears as a red rash on a person's skin, but with dogs we only see a loss of hair (alopecia). This can be anywhere on the dog's body, but usually is seen on the sides. We see this more often in younger dogs; probably because their immune systems are not yet fully developed to defend against these invaders from outer space.

Both types of mange are caused by tiny mites. The sarcoptic mites burrow under the skin much like a mole does under a lawn. The demodectic mites choose to drill down to the base of the hair follicles. Thusly, both kinds cause the loss of hair.

The sarcoptic mites are easily taken away by weekly doses of Ivermectin. Usually, three or four of these doses will do the trick, but let your veterinarian have the final word.

2. Demodectic

Demodectic mites first present an area that I liken to a "moth-eaten" fur coat. These spots can appear anywhere on the body. There may be one spot on a shoulder, another on the cheek, another on the side, etc. The only method by which we can positively identify these little critters is by performing a skin scraping, and then examining what we scrape under the microscope.

The demodectic mites are more difficult to annihilate. For just one or two small areas, the doctor may prescribe Goodwinol ointment, which must be rubbed in daily for weeks. If there are multiple areas, a very potent dip solution may also be used at weekly intervals, either with or without Goodwinol ointment.

The vast majority of demodectic cases will be cured. I'm sad to say, there are some young dogs that contract demodectic mange as small puppies, and "refuse to be cured". I have seen this occasionally. The owner would be very diligent in following all instructions. The puppy will get better, then worse. He will show improvement again, and then relapse. After many months of this, the owner will throw in the towel and say, "Enough is enough— please put the pup to sleep!"

I consider this an immune system failure. Often, this same client will have had a litter mate with mange at the same time, and this puppy will respond to the treatment very successfully. All dogs are different!

G. Pyoderma

This is a bacterial infection of the skin. It can occur in small areas anywhere on the body or even encompass the entire body and legs. This latter situation is usually in puppies with very poor immunity. If pyoderma continues to grow in the skin, for a long time, a smelly, 'stinky feet' smell results (unlike the yeast smell) and it permeates the bedding, car, couch, etc.

There is treatment, but an owner must be very diligent to follow through on the veterinarian's instructions in order to effect a cure. Many times, puppies that have not responded well to treatment are euthanized. Fortunately, most cases of pyoderma do respond nicely to antibiotics, along with medicated shampoos. It is important to remember to destroy bedding that has been slept on by an infected dog.

Clean the new bedding regularly with a bleach solution to kill whatever bacteria that might be left living on the 'blankie' and toys.

CHAPTER NINE

REPRODUCTIVE ORGANS

Let the criticisms begin! You paid a lot of money for your female puppy, so you want to breed her for your enjoyment and sell the puppies for a handsome profit! Or, you, sir, have this majestic male pup and, since manhood is supposed to rule, only over your dead body will anybody dare to neuter your precious Bruno!

God forbid! Don't even entertain the thought! As he matures, if he chooses to run off for a few days because some neighbor's female dog is in heat, "That's okay, he's just doing what nature intended." And when your next-door neighbor has just washed and polished his nice car, it is okay for Bruno to pee all over his shiny wheels and tires. And when your wife, or someone else's, has just planted some prize petunias, again, it is fine for Bruno to help keep them watered!

I really disagree with your reasoning. If you fit into the above category, then please erect a solid, 10 foot high fence so you can enjoy Bruno full-time and no neighbor will have reason to dislike your canine testosterone factory. Statistically, neutered males live longer, healthier lives. If a male pup is neutered between four and six months of age, the owner will not have to be concerned about the above shenanigans. Not to mention, there will be no testicular or prostatic cancer to ever have to worry about. In addition, the neutered male, I believe, is a better full-time loving companion.

I recommend that female dogs be spayed (this is an ovariohysterctomy) no later than six months of age. Some owners will obtain a female puppy in order to breed her so the children can "learn about the miracle of birth" and enjoy the puppies; the real crying starts when the puppies go home with their new owners. After all, this has been an investment and owners will want the profits from the sale of the puppies!

A. Breeding (On purpose or not)

Most dogs will go into 'heat' at about eight months of age, some earlier. Larger dogs tend to be later in becoming 'ready'. It is ill advised to let a young bitch get bred. It is much akin to a young teen-aged girl becoming pregnant. Just because this is physiologically possible, does not mean it should be done.

Very frequently, oh, so often, when this young pup is in the middle of the heat period, which lasts for 21 days, one of the children will go running out of the house not closing the door completely. The half-grown nymph bolts out the door—gone in a flash! When the concerned owner realizes what has happened and begins searching, and calling, and calling, and driving around the neighborhood, and calling, and looks, and looks, for this wayward pup, she is finally found. But not like the family wanted to find her— she is breeding with the biggest, ugliest dog in the neighborhood! Now the damage has been done. "Maybe she won't conceive,", "What will happen if she does?", "What about the puppies?", "What about the profits?" Now, everyone is sorry. And the young female may be in real trouble.

The normal gestation period is 63 days, nine weeks. Mom and Dad look at a calendar—they had planned a family vacation just about that time. Oh, well, there is nothing to do but just wait. As the weeks go by, Sheba's abdomen enlarges. Her mammary glands develop. As the ninth week approaches, the family still wants to take their planned vacation. Perhaps they can put Sheba in a boarding kennel, and she can have her puppies there. (How thoughtful!)

The evening before they are supposed to leave on their trip, little Sheba goes into labor. Everyone waits to anxiously see what happens. As the hours go by, the young dog is experiencing pain and just not delivering. The family bundles her into the car for a trip to the emergency clinic. Many hours have now passed since labor first began. They surrender Sheba to the staff for an examination and digital x-rays.

After a short time, the staff veterinarian brings the bad news: there is a puppy, which is now dead, lodged in the pelvic canal and is too large to come out. There are six more puppies in the uterus. The only way to save them, and Sheba, is with a Cesarean operation. The owners realize there is no other choice, so they give their permission to proceed. When the husband asks for a ballpark estimate of all the costs and is given the answer, husband and wife, are shocked! The amount quoted was almost as much as they were going to spend on their family vacation!

While Sheba goes in to life saving, and possibly dangerous surgery, the parents explain their changed plans to the children. Since they cannot afford the trip and the surgery the only choice is to stay home with Sheba and her six gigantic pups. That is, if they all make it through the surgery.

The story continues: Sheba made it through the surgery with the six remaining pups, and is now home, but, the large pups take so much milk from Sheba that the family has to supplement bottle feeding these critters until they can begin taking baby food on their own. Since puppies eat every two hours or so, even the children are becoming tired of nursing these quickly growing creatures. The family is eagerly looking forward to the day they can find new homes for these four-legged King Kong's. Everyone has had their fill of puppy nursing.

Now, they have six mixed breed puppies that seem to take after their father more than their lovely mother. In other words, they are not very cute as puppies should be. How to find homes for them? (This is very much a part of responsible pet ownership). Oh well, there is always the local animal shelter. We can let them find new homes for all the ugly ducklings! (Again, how thoughtful)! How many would—be pets are euthanized every week, every month, year after year, because there are too many animals that are unwanted? This tale is not just fiction— I have seen this in real life, time and time again.

If you truly want to breed your female puppy, guard her with your life during that first heat, period, for a full three weeks. Usually, the second heat will follow in about six months. Already have your plans made with the owner of the intended stud. This is the only way to by-pass vacation plans going awry. So many owners will wait until Juliet is well into the second heat, and then scramble to find the proper stud dog, often to no avail.

Arrangements must be made. Does the male come to your house for a few hours, or does Juliet go to his house and yard (a completely new situation)? Has the timing been planned properly? All of these things must be thought through.

Beginning the day vaginal bleeding is first noted, even a few drops, this is counted as the first day of heat. Most females will ovulate between the tenth and fourteenth days of heat. This is obviously the most fertile time for breeding.

It is always wise to have two breedings if possible. I recommend that both owners be present, letting Romeo and Juliet get acquainted in the beginning (first date) on the tenth day. Ninety-nine times out of a hundred, she will snarl at Romeo and tell him to get lost in no uncertain terms!

So, you try them together the next day. If her attitude continues for the next few days, and just will not permit Romeo to mount her, then her owner has to muzzle her, and hold her still in order for the desired result to occur. Of course, plans had to be changed—someone had to take off from work, give up golf games, arrange rides from dance lessons, find another coach for soccer, etc. In one way or another, every member of the family is affected.

After all of this effort, Miss Juliet has refused to breed with the Romeo you had chosen. But, leave the door partly open, and she will be gone in a flash to meet the neighborhood Fonzie around the corner. He was her choice! One quick breeding is all it takes and, voilà, you have a basket of mixed, unwanted, no profit puppies.

Now, please understand, I am just describing, as a warning, dramas that very frequently occur in real life. There are, also, many happy breedings that come off without a hitch, and beautiful puppies are the result. A word of caution: Ms. Juliet will usually go back into heat six months from the previous one. Getting pregnant does not alter that. So, an owner should plan to have her spayed as soon as the pups are gone, and her mammary glands are much diminished. By this time, a good four months, plus, have passed and you want to have her operated well before six months. This is easier on her and the surgeon.

But, alas, the owner wants to breed her again. The last gestation wasn't really that much trouble and that owner certainly enjoyed the money when they sold those pups! (Even though owners, usually, hardly break even with the expenses involved!) Ah, the "puppy mill syndrome". The Maple Street Puppy Factory!

Do I sound cynical? I love cute little puppies. Invariably, with these dogs, Planned Parenthood goes amiss. "We did not intend for her to get bred again so soon! It just happened!".

B. Mammary Tumors

Very often, these perpetually producing females will never get spayed, resulting in mammary tumors (cancer) that will necessitate early surgical removal. It is best to remove these while they are still small and well before they have had a chance to metastasize. At this time, an ovariohysterectomy must be performed to remove the source of hormones that are causing the problem. These poor animals have to have breast removal surgery and a hysterectomy at the same time! Had they been spayed just before their first heat, or perhaps after their first litter, they would've never had to go through this. The average production rate for a puppy mill female will often be over 100 puppies! Too bad she was not just a beloved pet, but a means to an end, usually her own.

C. Pyometra

Another often seen condition in older intact females is pyometra. This is from an infection in the uterus that has produced a boat load of pus. The cervix is usually closed so the situation can become dire. This uterus becomes toxic with the infection and mess inside it, and will kill the patient unless an ovariohysterectomy is soon performed. How many times have I seen this in an emergency clinic on a weekend night!? Episodes like this just upset everyone's apple cart! The owner then becomes concerned about the cost, and family plans, etc. and lastly about the dog.

Ovariohysterectomy is major surgery. Although dogs seem to heal with superpowers, they still experience some pain, anxiousness, and discomfort. They will require bed-rest to heal, protection from other animals and children, and will need gentle compassion and assistance. If you are a woman and have had a hysterectomy, or other type of major surgery, I don't need to explain this to you. Just as with people, different dogs heal at different rates. Age, general health, and quality of care are all factors in success of healing.

D. Dystocia

A difficult delivery is termed a dystocia. So many owners of pregnant female dogs just expect their little mommies to do all nature intended with no problems. Perhaps most of the time, this is what occurs. But, not always!

For whatever reason, it seems like most about-to-be mothers begin their labor activities in the afternoon. By the time family members arrive home, they noticed that Daisy has been in the whelping box for a while, and appears uncomfortable.

So this is the day she's having her puppies! Now, any special plans for the evening have to be canceled. It is absolutely necessary to observe Daisy, closely, for labor contractions.

Take note of when they started, and how long do they last? As the hours go by, and anxiety sets in, decisions must be made. "Shouldn't we be seeing a puppy by now?" Fortunately, you were able to contact your veterinarian's office just as they were closing, and you were given the phone number to the local animal emergency clinic. You may have been advised that after Daisy began having steady contractions, a puppy should be produced within an hour. If the contractions continued longer, she is in big trouble.

At this stage, nothing is to be gained by waiting any longer. Getting Daisy to the emergency clinic is paramount. She will be examined, and x-rays made of her innards, and you would be advised as to how many puppies are present, their approximate size, and why the bottle neck preventing delivery of the first puppy.

By this time, the staff clinician will probably recommend doing an immediate Cesarean section. It must be done or the mommie and puppies will die. The "secret" to performing successful Caesarean sections is to do them early, before the poor little mama is exhausted (and her body extremely stressed) and the puppies have all died.

The bottleneck puppy may be dead, but the others may be all right and Daisy will, probably, make an uneventful recovery, if supported completely during healing.

So, dear reader, I am not trying to discourage you from canine reproduction. My intention is to inform you of all the possibilities that can and do take place in the canine physiological world, things not told you in the pet shop or at the kennel when you obtained your best friend.

I want to dissuade you from any selfish motives and persuade you to think of what is best for your friend's health and well-being. There are so many "old wives tales" that have been passed on from generation to generation that are just plain foolishness! Things like, "A female dog should go through her first heat before she is spayed", and, "Let her have a litter of puppies, she'll be a better pet." These are the statements of ill-informed people. Then again, there is no law against ignorance.

When you have any questions concerning your four-legged family member, consult with your veterinarian. Also, be aware that we are also human, and come in all kinds. Some think that they are God's gift to the animal world, and choose not to end their ego trip. But hopefully, there are enough of us that really desire to help animals, with a positive bedside manner, and human communication skills. If you haven't found a veterinarian that you and your dog like, keep looking. Ask friends and people that you meet with dogs. You may hear a name over and over that everyone says is a really caring vet.

I prefer the old-fashioned, small practice. The multiple doctor practice may be a necessary evil, but my main objection lies in the general function of administrating such a large business. If a client is needing to see his or her favorite veterinarian (in the group), and he or she is either all booked up or off on that particular day the result can be frustrating for the client. Also, with large practices, the multiple receptionists tend to lean towards impersonal service. When you are asked, "Have you been here before?", when you've been there thirty-two times in the last twelve years, somehow you just don't get a feeling of belonging. Something is missing. Where is the personal service of olden days?

Each of my practices was a solo adventure, so each staff member could easily remember most of the clients and their pets. Also, this opportunity to foster relationships with the pets and their owners contributed much towards a very pleasurable work day. And it was much easier for me to be able to develop a good bedside manner with my patients. It is a symbiotic relationship. To me, this is how professional reputations are developed. The ultimate compliment was paid me in my last practice when I was referred to as the "local James Heriot". Oh, that did make me feel special, and appreciated. We all need that!

CHAPTER TEN

INTERNAL ORGANS

A. The Heart

Some years ago I received a telephone call. The gentleman identified himself as a physician, and said he was listening to his dog's heart. He became alarmed when the heart skipped a beat. As he continued to listen, the heart skipped another beat. This was just too much for him! "What could this mean?" he asked.

His fears were allayed when I replied that this was quite normal; that dogs' tickers often skip a beat. It is of no consequence.

Congenital cardiac anomalies occur in puppies as with babies. But these are very infrequent, and can only be recognized by a veterinarian's listening to a puppy's heart with a stethoscope.

Cardiac problems arise in many dogs as they age just as in people. A great many of these can be helped and managed with medications, although some may not. How can we know which from which?

Prior to twenty-five years ago, the veterinary clinician only had his knowledge and best judgment with which to treat a dog with a heart problem. Otherwise, he would try to persuade the owner to transport his pooch to the nearest veterinary school to seek a cardiologist's expertise. But now we have veterinary cardiologists in larger cities.

There is no reason for the average practitioner to not refer the patient to a specialist, within a reasonable distance. Yes, it costs money, but its well worth it to get to the bottom of Fluffy's heart problem.

In performing an echocardiogram (an ultrasound of the heart), a good cardiologist, or internist, will be able to diagnose the problem, determine what treatment might help, and give a proper prognosis. All of this is invaluable, just as with humans. So, should your best friend undergo a cardiac episode, take heart! This is not a death sentence. Learn to pray, if you haven't already. Your beloved can enjoy many more years of normal life!

1. Heartworms

This topic is, without question, the single most important cause of premature cardiac malfunction in all the canine population in America. This has been the case for sixty-odd years that I know of, and probably much longer than that.

In about 1960, Norden Laboratories distributed a map to all small animal practitioners showing, geographically, the areas of natural heartworm infestation of dogs in America. Heartworms are transmitted only by mosquito bites. So, in the beginning, the affected areas were primarily the Ohio and Mississippi River valleys and the southeastern states. Every year this map has been updated to show the geographical spread of naturally occurring cases. For quite a number of years now, the map completely engulfs all of the United States!

This disease is so easily preventable. The oral heartworm preventive given monthly, at the proper dose, all year round, if started in puppy hood, is the guaranteed prevention. Adult dogs will need to be tested for heartworms before any preventative is given. This must be done with your veterinarian's direction.

Unfortunately, too many owners try to cut corners in order to save a few bucks. They will second guess the weather just because they haven't seen any mosquitoes, they may skip Yellow Dawg's tablet this month, and completely forget it next month, etc.

In my book, the Yankee veterinarians in the northern states are playing Russian roulette with their clients' dogs by only recommending giving the preventive in the summer months. Hey, you guys, why are you still seeing heartworm infection? Oh, I know, your clients will not give it year round.

O.K., so, do you treat many of the infected dogs? Most of them survive the Immiticide treatment, right? And, do the owners find that expensive? It is a whole lot safer and cheaper to give the preventive all year round, regardless of where you live or the weather. A word to the wise should be sufficient!

B. The Lungs

It is necessary to continue our discourse on heartworms because of the damage to the lungs that occurs in just weeks of the worms becoming mature. Heartworms most closely resemble spaghetti in color, diameter, not nearly as much in length. Their first location is the pulmonary artery. As the worm burden increases, the right atrium, (or auricle) is the second campsite. As their number increases to about one hundred, they begin to obstruct the anterior vena cava (the large vein returning to the heart).

After a positive blood test is found, one of the first things done in diagnostics is to take x-rays of the chest. If the pulmonary artery appears enlarged and the heart shadow is wider, the clinician will proffer the bad news.

At this point, the pooch may not be showing any outward signs, like heavy breathing or tiring out on long walks. But, again he may just be beginning these. If this should be your dog, PLEASE follow your veterinarian's instructions to the letter. If so, your dog will probably come out perfectly all right. But follow the instructions all the way through.

Some years ago I treated a gorgeous Pointer, a field trial champion, for heartworms. The treatment was successful, but as the heartworms were killed, they began to disintegrate into small "foreign bodies". As these progressed, the blood circulation carried them into the arterioles of the small areas of the lungs, effectively obstructing circulation, resulting in pneumonic areas.

The dog was fine until he became excited, like going hunting, and then would start coughing. So instead of being able to point a covey of birds, he'd scare the whole field away with his coughing. Thus, he was quite useless from then on as a bird dog. I felt sorry for the owner, who was quite upset. But now, we have the preventative: give it!

1. Bronchitis

Commonly referred to as "kennel cough", this is a frequent malady of boarded dogs and those coming in close contact with others, such as doggy day care and dog parks. Actually, any place where dogs can "nose to nose" or breathe the same air.

All boarding kennels require dogs to be vaccinated against this. The Bordetella is not a vaccine but a bacterin, and needs to be repeated every six months. Even so, it is not 100% effective as a preventative. But if given at least two weeks before leaving FiFi that is the best for which you can hope.

A modern alternative to boarding is to hire a pet sitter. They come to your home and give your pet undivided love and attention in their own space. Yes, it may cost a little more (perhaps not), but would be worth it since other tasks could be performed such as: mail and newspapers will be brought in, your plants watered, lights turned on and off periodically, your dog walked and your house looks as if someone is home. It is an invaluable convenience. Your veterinarian probably has names of persons in your area and a reliable pet sitter should have good references.

The average case of bronchitis will last for ten to fourteen days, even with antibiotics. This infection is highly contagious to other dogs that are unvaccinated. There is a procedure that some vets may use to alleviate the symptoms. This is the injection of half antibiotic (Gentamycin) and half steroid administered directly into the trachea. Sometimes the results are seen the same day. Not every clinician may be familiar with this injection, so please have mercy. Remember we are all "practicing".

2. Canine Influenza

Now, we have the canine flu with which to contend. There is a vaccine available through your veterinarian, and this needs to be repeated periodically. The symptoms for canine flu include temperature elevated, even when not so active, increased respiration, and lack of appetite. The treatment is usually aimed at relieving the symptoms. Since this is a viral infection, antibiotics are of little value.

3. Collapsed Trachea

This is not an unusual condition of small dogs, like small Poodles, Maltese, Yorkies, and other toy breeds. The cause is unknown. For whatever reason, a portion of the trachea, in the chest, just closes down to maybe half its normal diameter. Only a portion of the trachea is affected, maybe two to three inches of the middle.

This is easily seen and diagnosed by x-ray. Usually the only sign the owner notices is an unusual cough, unlike any other. Looking at an x-ray of the average collapsed trachea, I have said to myself a number of times, "There must be a way to surgically correct this." Veterinary textbooks describe a couple of methods of repair.

After postulating my own ideas, I have discussed these with surgeons who assure me others have tried similar techniques, none with success. The mechanics of a corrective procedure should not appear to be that difficult, nevertheless better surgeons than I, have tried several techniques, but none have been successful. I know not why. Hopefully, someone will keep trying until they do find a successful method of helping these poor little dogs.

4. Second-hand cigarette smoke

I don't know why I even have to mention this. Surely, all dog owners are intelligent enough to know NO ONE CAN BE ALLOWED TO SMOKE IN THE SAME HOUSE OR CAR, with a dog, children, another man's wife, or anyone! Scientific study after scientific study has shown proof of the harm of second-hand cigarette smoke. With dogs, besides lung cancer, emphysema is the most common condition seen. There are medications that might help to a certain extent, but, as in humans, there is no cure.

C. Stomach

Allow me a general observation: dogs are able to vomit very easily, almost at will, it seems. We two-legged beings immediately think something terrible is taking place in precious pooch's innards. But, probably 90% of the time, there is no cause for alarm. The other 10% is when there are other accompanying signs, such as bad diarrhea, and obviously feeling poorly.

This occurs when Caesar has been fed bones (any kind of bones!) or invaded the garbage bag. Your veterinarian needs to make the decision on the possible seriousness of the situation. Which brings to mind another story: in my first practice, one morning the phone rang. As I answered it, this lady was yelling and crying. I could hear what sounded like a child screaming in pain in the background. I could only understand her when she said her name. I hastily pulled her record, saw her address was about a mile away, grabbed my medical bag and jumped into my car. Ignoring all traffic laws, I arrived at her apartment building, bounded up the stairs, and burst through her door. This poor woman was on her knees, bent over the lifeless body of her little white Poodle, just crying her heart out. In between sobs, she explained what had transpired. Her husband had taken her little dog out to "do his business" before he left for work. Shortly thereafter, the miniature poodle had begun showing signs of discomfort. As these worsened, she phoned me. They had no children. What I had thought was a child screaming in pain, was actually this poor little dog. Then he died.

After some time, this lady regained her composure, and I suggested my taking her beloved back with me, to do an autopsy. She agreed. In performing the procedure, I found only chicken bones, from the stomach into a good portion of the small intestine. It was each of these sharp bones, raking into the intestinal wall that had caused the severe pain, internal bleeding, and then death!

When I reported this to the owner, she could not understand where her poodle obtained the chicken bones. Later, she rang me back after conferring with her husband, to say the poor beast had poked his head very quickly into the neighbor's open garbage bag, as the husband was about to take him out that morning. Just long enough for him to consume a lethal load of chicken bones I have seen so many problems over the years from all kinds of bones— big and little, sharp and smooth— so my admonition to all dog lovers is, never give your dog any kind of bones! Period!

Dogs are carnivores, yes, their digestive enzymes are supposed to assimilate meat; however, they cannot digest bones. These only act as foreign bodies, and are of no benefit whatsoever! Wild dogs DO make the required enzymes to digest bones. Modern, domestic dogs do not have these enzymes produced naturally in their bodies.

John Bloxham, D.V.M.

Besides indigestion and vomiting from unusual food, the next most serious condition is the result of poor Fido not being able to regurgitate, burp, or help himself to relieve stomach gases.

1. Gastric dilatation-volvulus (GDV)

GDV can be the nightmare of all stomach problems of large dogs—from Pointers to St. Bernards, from Irish Setters to Great Danes, and all breeds in between. This is an acute, life-threatening disorder that is a medical and surgical emergency. Even with early recognition and treatment, less than half of the affected dogs come through with flying colors. This less than desirable survival rate is due to all of the complicating factors of GDV, and should not be a reflection of the care rendered by any medical personnel.

A dilated stomach may or may not be accompanied by volvulus—a twisting of the stomach that completely obstructs any outflow to the intestines, or vomiting or belching, to relieve the rapid accumulation of fluid and gas. When this does occur, massive distention of the stomach blocks venous circulation, causing endo-toxic shock.

Congestion of the abdominal viscera predisposes to chemical imbalance, affecting the blood. The spleen may be displaced with problems of its' own. A portion of the stomach wall may become necrotic. All of these factors contribute to a very guarded prognosis of GDV when presented to any emergency clinic.

A definitive cause is unknown. Several theories have been promulgated over the years but none proven. Swallowed air is believed to be a factor, such as gulping one's food. Over-eating, exercise after eating, and dry food have been suggested to predispose to GDV, but none of these have been substantiated clinically or experimentally.

Probably the first symptom the owner will notice is his/her pet is very uncomfortable and restless. Dogs are very stoic—as they don't readily complain of pain. But with GDV, the dog has a severe bellyache, and the stomach is becoming more and more distended. This usually occurs within a few hours of the dog's having been fed, so the vast majority of these cases will be seen in the evening at emergency clinics. Yes, this is expensive, but your dog will die a very painful death if untreated.

I have seen a few of these conditions in the morning, and one Irish Setter at 2 PM, but most occur in the evening. Some doctors will recommend several smaller feedings during the day in hopes of preventing GDV. So follow your veterinarian's recommendations, and not on Dr. Google.

I strongly recommend dogs that have survived a bout of GDV not be boarded. You do not want to change any environmental or eating habit factors. Hire that pet sitter to stay at your home and follow your exact instructions. A good pet sitter is worth her weight in gold! Just ask your dog when you return from a trip!

D. The Liver

The liver is the largest internal organ, and has at least twenty-one functions; no beast can live without a healthy liver. There are numerous causes of liver dysfunction, really too many to enumerate here.

Whenever a veterinarian draws blood during the annual exam for a "full panel", this will include three or four liver enzyme function tests. These are very important, and readily reveal if Maggie's liver might be impaired. For dogs that are on NSAIDs, such as Rimadyl, for arthritic pain, these liver enzymes should be checked even more frequently. It is recommended that every 3 to 6 months to check for any changes that may have occurred. We all have heard of horror stories from people whose dogs were started on Rimadyl, then got very sick and died within a few days. These happen, just like with human drugs, albeit rare in number. Any elevated liver enzyme can sound an alarm but do not pin point liver dysfunction.

There are other tests, such as serum bile acid concentrations and others, that are more definitive for liver disease. Should your pet be so unfortunate as to develop an hepatic disease, I would hope your veterinarian would refer you to an internist (if one is available in your area). The reason being, that any disease of the liver can be so complicated, and will affect other organs. This is my opinion and best advice.

E. The Pancreas

1. Diabetes

Although not nearly as prevalent as in the human population, diabetes does occur in the canine kingdom. I will not go into the usual symptoms, because I don't want owners to start guessing. Any time your pooch seems "not quite right" is the perfect time to visit your veterinarian.

Allow him/her to do diagnostic blood testing— this eliminates so much guesswork. If the problem should be diabetes, a blood glucose test readily proves this. Then your veterinarian will thoroughly discuss the entire treatment regimen with insulin.

2. Pancreatitis

This is an acute condition with poorly understood ramifications. In most dogs with spontaneous pancreatitis, the cause cannot be identified. We do know that the pancreatic enzymes become out of balance.

The most common symptoms are vomiting, not eating, depression, and dehydration. There will be pain in the abdomen over the pancreas and diarrhea (perhaps bloody). These signs are accompanied by fever and weakness. This dog is sick, sick, sick!

You must seek immediate help, and don't bother to ask what treatment will cost. At this point nobody knows or can tell you. This treatment constitutes critical care. There is no single treatment for pancreatitis. Everything will sound complicated and drawn out, but is absolutely necessary. The vast majority of these patients experience a good recovery, if all the treatment protocol is prompt and followed through.

F. The Kidneys

As dogs age, their kidneys can begin to show "wear and tear", especially if a patient's blood pressure has been elevated (hypertension) over a period of time.

Someone of authority stated years ago, that any dog's kidneys can function all right on as little as 25% of normal kidney tubules. But if anything alters that 25% figure to reduce it in the slightest, that pooch will suffer symptoms of kidney (renal) failure. I don't know how accurate that statement may still be.

The two universal blood tests that are used to determine kidney function are blood urea nitrogen and creatinine. The first test (BUN) measures the amount of waste material the kidneys are able to excrete from the body. The creatinine measures the kidneys ability to excrete the waste material. The numerical value given in the creatinine test is exponential. That is, if a patient's creatinine is two one day, and three the next, this is twice as bad. If it is four the next day, that is twice as bad as the day before, and so forth. Thus when treating a dog for kidney failure, we can keep tabs on the progress of the therapy, or lack thereof.

One note of encouragement: acute renal failure is a potentially reversible condition. This will necessitate 24 hour intravenous fluid therapy (in a hospital— no you cannot take him home!) for a duration of seven to fourteen days. If the treatments are done properly, this should result in Harley's complete recovery.

The $64 question: what caused this? Acute nephritis is usually caused by infection. Another of the most common causes is a dogs lapping some anti-freeze spilled in a driveway. The ethylene glycol in anti-freeze has a sweet taste but is deadly. Aspirin and ibuprofen have also been incriminated, but we know better than to give these to our pets, don't we?

With any type of kidney disease, prompt and thorough treatment is paramount to a successful outcome. This includes hustling to an emergency clinic at night rather than waiting until morning to go to your regular veterinarian for a drop off. By the time they would get any labs done, twelve more hours of damage will have been accomplished, and any treatment delayed that much longer.

Chronic renal failure occurs most often in older creatures. If there is a good veterinary internist nearby (within 100 miles) a referral to this doctor could prove invaluable to your gaining knowledge of what is going on with your pet's urinary system, and perhaps the outcome. The prognosis may still be guarded, but you will have a better understanding of why this is happening, etc.

Your veterinarian should be able to keep tabs on the patient's blood pressure. Systolic pressure greater than 180 and diastolic pressure greater than 95mm mercury means hypertension. As with humans, this causes over-load in the kidneys, and will be detrimental over time. To help manage hypertension, dietary sodium restriction is the initial step. Your pet's doctor can recommend a special food for this.

G. Urinary Bladder

In everyday practice, the two most common problems seen involving the bladder are urinary calculi (or bladder stones) and bacterial infections. A diagnosis of cystitis just means inflammation of the urinary bladder, by any cause.

1. Urinary Calculi

There are half a dozen types of urinary calculi, based on their mineral composition. But the one most commonly seen in dogs is of magnesium ammonium phosphate. When a dog is urinating only a small amount frequently, and especially if any blood is seen, bladder stones may be suspected as one of the causes of the cystitis. Your veterinarian will need to perform a urinalysis and get x-rays of the bladder. There may be one large stone, but more frequently there are a bunch of them in various sizes.

Many times, these can be dissolved by putting Goldie on a special diet for at least a month, then do another pair of x-rays to determine the progress. For the dogs that are really having difficulty urinating (dysuria), I recommend prompt surgery—a cystotomy, to open the bladder and physically remove all of the stones. If done properly, and effective medicines used, the dog should have uncomplicated recovery. Then diet can be discussed to, hopefully, prevent reoccurrence.

2. Bacterial Infections

Bacterial infections of the urinary tract can be very complicated, and I don't mean to simplify this very common cause. This is why a urinalysis is paramount for diagnostics including bacterial cultures and sensitivity tests. Frequently an antibiotic will be given that may annihilate one bacteria, but not affect another. So then, a different antibiotic must be used. After a few weeks, your veterinarian will want to check another urinalysis with cultures to be certain the problem is licked. Otherwise, Felicia will just keep licking.

Whenever a diagnosis of bacterial cystitis is given to an owner, there is always the question, "How did he get this?!" My stock answer for many years has been, "If you go to a urologist's office, there are people sitting there with the same problem as your dog. They bathe every day, put on clean underwear daily, never sit on the floor or ground naked, and do not lick themselves! I don't know how they get their infections, but I'm never surprised to see it in dogs!"

3. Tumors of the Bladder

a. Transitional Cell Carcinoma

Although not seen too frequently, we do need to mention tumors of the bladder: these are usually malignant and more common in female dogs and tend to occur in older dogs about ten years of age. One of the most common cancers is transitional cell carcinoma. This monster usually shows up near the neck of the bladder. Unfortunately, there is no satisfactory treatment for its demise, surgery or otherwise.

Years ago, I was working at the North Charleston, South Carolina emergency clinic for a few months. One night a lady brought in a white, miniature poodle with the main symptom of "A.D.R." Now, she didn't use this term—this is only used among clinic personnel to explain a patient's problem. This term is somewhat precise, more or less. These three letters stand for "Ain't Doing Right". There may not be any specific signs you can point to, so you have to look deeper.

With this little doggie, a female, the owner mentioned that she had been spayed at a nearby hospital three or four days before and just hadn't been herself since. She was sick; not eating and just listless. My lightning fast mind immediately decided that there was something amiss from the surgery. I explained this to the lady, and sought permission to anesthetize the sick poodle in order to do exploratory surgery. She agreed and left her with me.

I anesthetized the little dog, undid all of the spay sutures, and was shocked to see she had no urinary bladder! It was gone! Apparently, when the surgeon (?!) removed the uterus, he included the bladder with it! So, the two ureters, from the kidneys, were just dumping their urine in the abdominal cavity. I went to the phone to call the vet who supposedly had performed the spay operation, and he immediately came over to see for himself. He appeared as surprised as I was. The poor little dog was already becoming toxic from the uremia, so I had to euthanize her. Needless to say, the lady was very distraught. I don't know what transpired between her and the other vet. None of us like to talk about our mistakes.

4. Urinary Incontinence

These cases are most commonly seen in older, spayed female dogs. They will dribble urine when relaxed or asleep. They do not mean to do it, and feel quite ashamed when they awaken to find their rear ends in a puddle of urine. They do not need to be scolded, they need to be loved and pitied.

Trot yourself down to your local veterinary office, and ask for a bottle of "PPO tablets". These are Phenylpropanalamine, and are tasty and chewable. These tablets have to be given daily for the rest of Maggie's life.

These tablets usually solve the problem nicely, as long as they are given daily. This urinary disorder is caused by a lack of female hormones. Some authorities want to blame very early ovariohysterectomy (8 to 12 weeks of age) as the cause of incontinence later. As much as I disapprove of pediatric spays, I don't think that this theory holds water.

CHAPTER ELEVEN

INFECTIOUS DISEASES

A. Parvovirus

We shouldn't have to be concerned with this topic, IF every dog owner would have his/her pet properly vaccinated, beginning at an early age and continuing to the cemetery. But, unfortunately, some puppies are sold from "backyard breeders" as having had "some shots" or "first shots" or "all shots" with no documentation. The unwary buyer is lulled into thinking the pup is all right and there is no need to seek an animal pediatrician for a proper examination and anything else that cute little thing may need. Never mind the need for deworming.

This scenario occurs again and again, and this is the main reason we are still seeing so much parvo virus. This nightmare of infection first hit in America, in 1979 in the New York area from Europe. Until then, it was an unheard of disease here.

It spread across the country to California, then back east-ward through southern states to Florida, and then raged up the east coast, arriving in Virginia early summer of 1980.

This was, and is, a very devastating disease. Entire litters, often including the mothers, were wiped out. We had no vaccine against it. The pharmaceutical companies worked feverishly to develop a parvo vaccine. So finally they did, and in large enough quantities to serve the whole country.

I always advised breeding mothers to be 'boostered' (another series of injections) before they are bred. This should provide protection to puppies as long as they are nursing. And immediately at this point, the puppies should be vaccinated and the vaccine repeated in two weeks. When the kids go to new homes, give some kind of documentation, to remind the new parents to continue these immunizations every two to three weeks. Let their veterinarian dictate the protocol.

For the folks who have proudly raised a litter to eight weeks of age, and now you are advertising them, let me play the role of a concerned parent: A car drives up, an entire family comes to your door to announce they've come to see your puppies! You open wide the door and in your mind you see dollar signs. Both parents and each of the children hold and hug every puppy. As the children are saying that they each want a different one, the parents let slip that they probably can't afford one right now, because they still owe the emergency clinic almost a thousand dollars for trying to save their last puppy with parvo, just a few days ago.

Now, do you see in your haste to make some money, you have just exposed all of your puppies to parvo virus? Since ten days are required for a vaccine to begin to provide immunity, your pups may not be all right.

Parvo virus has a short incubation period, only five days from exposure. The first symptoms seen are profuse vomiting and diarrhea. With this the pup feels badly, is very depressed, and hurting because the virus is actually destroying the lining of the intestines. Any treatment must be prompt and critical. This means 24 hour intravenous drips of various fluids with nutrients since the patient is unable to eat. This critical care must be continued for at least 4, 5, 6 or more days until the symptoms are vastly improved and one can assume the danger is over.

It is impossible to guess which pup will pull through and which one will not. We have all seen young dogs come in with parvo that are caught early and don't seem to be very bad. We veterinarians are inclined to give the owner a hopeful prognosis with the statement, "I think he'll be okay in three or four days."

Sometimes, if we say this, that will be the pup who is really doing badly in 3 or 4 days, and may not survive. Conversely, we see puppies come into the hospital that have been sick for 2 or 3 days, look and feel terrible, and many of these do survive with proper intense treatment.

All owners get the lecture about protective vaccinations from here on. After they've paid their big bill, they realize they've learned a valuable lesson.

B. Canine Distemper

The distribution of canine distemper is worldwide. It can affect all ages of unvaccinated dogs, but the highest incidence is in puppies. Affected dogs are really sick: they stop eating, have high fevers, purulent ocular and nasal discharges, pneumonia with cough, abdominal pustules, and at some point, central nervous system signs will develop. The virus hones in on the brain. All other symptoms are from secondary infections, and will respond to treatment. If a dog seems to recover, very soon he will either go into convulsions, or develop an involuntary muscle twitch in a fore leg, called "chorea". It is referred to as 'St. Vitus' Dance' in humans. There is no treatment.

For many, many years, distemper was the number one killer of dogs. It has now been replaced by parvo virus. The vast majority of veterinarians in practice today have never seen a single case of distemper, and may never get to. Why? Because for so many decades we preached and we preached annual vaccinations. When I was a young doctor, I saw hundreds and hundreds of canine distemper cases. If we didn't see one for a week, we would have two the next week. This was how prevalent it was. Thanks to the regular vaccinations given over the years, distemper is virtually unseen today. One could assume that it has been mostly eradicated. Hopefully, it won't make a comeback with the new three year protocol on some vaccines.

For the last few years, the annual vaccines have been superseded with the three year vaccines. They are supposed to provide the same efficacy of protection, only for a longer period. In all of my years of practice, I knew I would not get 100% of the owners coming back each year, no matter how many post cards we sent as reminders. (I could never figure why). I don't mean those who moved away, or were divorced, or whose pets died, I mean a whole bunch of good, sort-of regular clients who, for whatever reason, just chose not to come in for their pets' annual exam, fecal check, and heartworm test. And now we still expect them to come in hopefully every six months for a health exam, but definitely every three years for the vaccination booster. A large percentage of them will think, "Well, if it's good for three years, then why not three and a half or four?" So, I predict that we will see an increase in parvo cases, heartworm cases, internal parasites, and other health problems simply because of the newer three year protocol. I do hope that I'm wrong.

We have been using a three year rabies vaccine for many decades. But the dog owner is given a dated certificate and needs this to purchase a dog license. This is a good motivator for a reminder.

C. Canine Hepatitis

This is not the hepatitis disease that affects humans. As with distemper, we hear very little about it because the canine hepatitis vaccine has been incorporated with the canine distemper vaccine for the last 55 years. Here again, just keep your fuzzy friend properly vaccinated (early on and throughout) and you'll not need to be concerned with canine hepatitis.

D. Rabies Virus

With the development of the first avianized vaccine back in the early 1950's, we don't have the rabies epidemics that used to be so prevalent when I was young. At my first job in a veterinary hospital, I was bitten twice in one week by rabid dogs, but only had to take the series of vaccines one time. I survived.

Just for nomenclature, when dogs are showing signs of rabies, we speak of two types – dumb and furious. (No, I don't mean the veterinarian!).

When an owner first suspects something amiss, a rabid dog's personality becomes the opposite. He doesn't respond to commands, doesn't know where he is or who you are. He will readily bite or attack any other dog without provocation. There is no question of something affecting the brain.

Their throats become paralyzed, so they cannot eat or drink, even though they try. The tongue hangs out, collecting dirt with saliva. It is a pitiful sight indeed. Nearly always the rabid dog will die within just two or three days of this stage. Then the health department wants us to decapitate the poor critter so they can submit the brain to their lab for positive diagnosis. What an end! A bad day for everyone!

E. Lyme's Disease

This is a disease that affects man and beast. It was named for Lyme, Connecticut; I suppose someone there first contracted it. This is transmitted by ticks. The deer tick is the one usually accused of being the culprit, but other ticks also can spread the disease. Many dogs do not show any symptoms with Lyme's; these are found by a positive blood test. The most common symptom observed is lameness that may shift from one leg to another.

Whenever there is a positive test, antibiotics are recommended for at least three weeks. Doxycycline is the one of choice.

F. Leptospirosis

This disease is more common than most people realize. If there is a three-year vaccine for this, I do not know it. Fort Dodge just a few years ago, was improving their preparations, but only for annual vaccinations. Leptospirosis would be expected to be anywhere dogs urinate – kennels, day care centers, doggie parks, etc. The organism, a spirochete, is spread through urine. Humans are often exposed from rats and mice contaminating tabletops and eating utensils.

Symptoms in dogs can be fever, not eating, depression, acute renal failure, even liver failure. The other bad news is that this is difficult to diagnose, and can only be proven by laboratory results that take time to accomplish.

Some years ago, a high school boy in New Jersey got a summer job in an animal hospital. He began on Monday morning. Within a couple of days, he had become sick and went to a physician who sent him to the local hospital. His condition worsened rapidly, and by the weekend, he had died. After all the tests and lab work had been completed, the diagnosis was leptospirosis!

Yes, we all know of bad things that happened to good people. But let's not forget the good things that happen in the lives of good people and good dogs.

CHAPTER TWELVE

INTERNAL PARASITES

A. Coccidiosis

This is a condition only seen in new puppies. Coccidia are only seen under the microscope on a fecal smear. These parasites are caused by dirty surroundings while pups are still with mom. The main symptom is diarrhea, maybe watery.

Fortunately, this is a self-limiting infection after the puppy is removed from the old environment. Your veterinarian can give you either tablets or a liquid to help stop the diarrhea and speed recovery.

B. Roundworms

These are the most common internal parasites of any puppy and most dogs. Puppies get them from their mothers and grown dogs from contaminated soil. The treatment is very simple. Most of the monthly heartworm preventatives also will prevent roundworms and hookworms.

C. Hookworms

Hookworms are almost as common as roundworms, and also obtained from mother and contaminated ground. They bite into the intestinal wall and suck blood. They can cause bloody diarrhea in young dogs. They are also easily treated.

D. Whipworms

These are only seen in mature dogs, usually confined to a fenced yard. The most common sign noticed by an owner is blackish diarrhea. **Whipworms** inhabit the lower large intestine, and sometimes treatment is not fully successful. Also if the pooch is returned to the same contaminated yard, he may easily become re-infected. Frequent fecal exams would be recommended to be certain a cure has been effected.

E. Tapeworms

This is the only internal parasite we diagnose by seeing— grossly. They look like flat grains of rice either on a bowel movement or lying in the hair beside the rectum. What we see are segments of an adult **tapeworm**, still lodged in the intestines. These segments contain the tapeworm eggs. As these segments dry out and begin to disintegrate, a flea will come by and swallow some of these tapeworm eggs. When the flea jumps on a dog the dog chews his fur and swallows the flea thus completing the cycle. Dogs can only get tapeworms from swallowing the contaminated fleas. So in addition to giving medication to annihilate the tapeworms, we also have to counsel the owner concerning flea control for immediate application.

F. Heartworms

Heartworms are discussed in Chapter 10: Internal Organs, and is mentioned under Heart and Lungs.

DR. JACK'S THIS AND THAT

All of my life I have heard that dogs possess a certain "sixth sense". I suppose that the majority of dog keepers would quickly respond, "Mine does!" If asked for some proof of making that statement, a plethora of answers would all exclaim how smart he or she is, and the undeniable fact that the beloved in question is almost human! No one in his right mind would dare to argue with that level of reasoning! God forbid!

However, since God did create dogs (and all animals) for His pleasure as well as ours, we can assume that there are varying levels of intelligence, just as with humans. Could this mean that only the smarter canines would be endowed with that sixth sense? Or do all dogs possess this? I wish I could answer that.

Unfortunately, I'm only an observer and student of these marvelous animals, but I have learned much from them. Allow me to elaborate: we did a fair amount of boarding dogs at one of my hospitals. A family pet would be dropped off on a Monday morning to be boarded for a week. For six days this dog would be calm and quiet. At about 10 o'clock on the seventh day, this sedate pooch would begin to whine and yelp. This would continue for most of the day.

Finally, maybe about four or five in the afternoon, the owners would come to bail out their fuzzy critter. I asked them what time did they get back to town. They would reply, "We got home about ten this morning but we had a lot of things to do, so this is why we are late getting here". I have witnessed occurrences like this, innumerable times over the years.

On a personal note, when I came to Richmond, Virginia in the latter 1950s, my best friend was Buster, an adorable tan and white Cocker spaniel. He was with me during the last two years in vet school. I took him to classes with me, until the day a clumsy professor stepped on his ear. After that episode, he agreed to stay in the small animal clinic where he lived with me.

Anyway, fast forward to Richmond four years later; I would drive home about 5 PM weekdays from the hospital where I was working and Buster would always sit on our front porch awaiting my coming. When my light blue Plymouth turned the corner, two blocks away, I could see that dog start jumping! That boy would come alive! He acted like I'd been away for a month. Such a tremendous welcome, on a daily basis! Every man should be so blessed.

It is said that dogs are color blind – not so! They may not see colors as vividly as we do, but they certainly can recognize shades of colors. My beloved friend always recognized my blue car, and also knew when I was to come home. And he didn't have a wristwatch! Don't try to tell me that dogs are not smart.

Sadly, about two years later, at age nine, my best friend developed Hodgkin's disease. Every lymph gland in his body became enlarged. Day by day, he grew more anemic. I gave him a blood transfusion, but he did not enjoy the procedure at all. Finally, when the day arrived that I did not think he was enjoying life, I made the fateful decision for him, and told him I'll be with him again in heaven.

It behooves me to make a comment here: every dog (all animals) has a body and a soul. The dog does not possess a spirit (only humans do) to be separated from God. We know the body decays after death, but the soul (the mind, the will, and the emotions) goes to heaven. How do I know this? There are a number of published works of people who have had "near death" experiences, some for only a few minutes to one who was in heaven for 90 minutes! These were folks who died from heart attacks, car wrecks and in surgery. All were prayed back to life.

Needless to say, their writings make for extremely interesting reading. A number of these who have been to heaven and returned, naturally spoke with friends and relatives who had gone on before. But some of these also reported their pet dogs, many of which had died years and years ago, came bounding up to greet them, in healthy bodies!

John Bloxham, D.V.M.

The Bible tells us that we two-legged animals will take on "glorified bodies" in which our spirits and souls will live forever. Apparently, the same holds for our four-legged friends. This is why I can boldly tell an owner whose dog has just succumbed, "The next time you see Beau, he won't be sickly or lame. He'll be running around in a young, healthy body."

Which brings up another point: every veterinarian is asked a common question, "At what point shall I put my dog to sleep? I don't want to be selfish and I don't want him to suffer".

My response is always the same: take one day at a time. If Goldie is eating and wagging her tail, and you think she is enjoying life today, then enjoy her. But the day you think she is not enjoying life, that is the day to end it.

Early one summer, years ago, our beloved Miniature Schnauzer, Brummel, took sick. Strange symptoms with no definite clues; I was baffled. I took my precious dog to a colleague for help. There was none forthcoming. He was just as baffled.

Since he wasn't eating, I had intravenous drips going into his veins at home. I only knew to give him supportive treatment. We didn't have all of the sophisticated laboratory testing available at that time, like we do now. Also, this was before the advent of board-certified specialists.

Needless to say, my wife and I were extremely concerned for our Brummel. His condition was worsening daily. We prayed for him, seemingly with no improvement. At this time a family who had been living in Germany for the past year stopped by to visit. We explained to them our great concern about Brummel. The husband said, "Let's pray for him!" So the four of us joined hands in a circle, and my friend prayed a very simple prayer for Brummel. After a short visit, they left.

My attention returned to Brummel. I had previously opened a can of smelly cat food, dipping one finger in and trying to coax him into licking it off my finger. Now, he not only licked my finger, he stuck his nose in the can, licking it clean! He began to drink water. I opened a can of dog food, and he readily consumed that. Needless to say, he continued to make a complete recovery, and enjoyed a healthy life for three more years after that.

I still have no idea what the underlying cause was of that illness, but I do know there is a God in heaven who answers prayer! A number of miracles have transpired in my life – in cats, dogs, people, and one young cow in Africa. But that must be another book for another day.

In His Majesty's service,
John C. Bloxham, DVM
A.K.A. Dr. Jack

www.ingramcontent.com/pod-product-compliance
Lightning Source LLC
Chambersburg PA
CBHW021005180526
45163CB00005B/1905